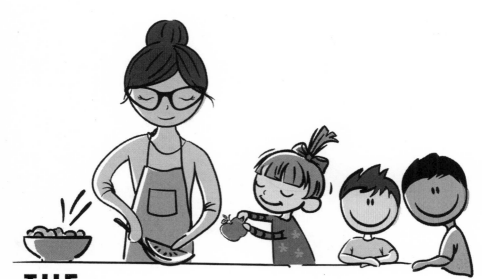

THE
SMART MOM'S
GUIDE
TO HEALTHY SNACKING

**How to Raise a Smart Snacker
from Tot to Teen**

JILL CASTLE

THE SMART MOM'S GUIDE TO HEALTHY SNACKING

HOW TO RAISE A SMART SNACKER FROM TOT TO TEEN

JILL CASTLE

NOURISHED CHILD PRESS

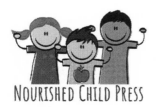

NOURISHED CHILD PRESS

CONTENTS

INTRODUCTION

I stood in the kitchen preparing dinner one night as my child came in and opened the pantry. She grabbed a box of crackers. I said, *"What are you doing? We're having dinner soon."*

"But I'm hungry now, Mom. Can't I just have a few?" she asked.

I felt my blood simmer.

Why am I putting all this effort into making a nice dinner, only for my daughter to ruin her appetite with a snack? I thought.

If I'm to be perfectly honest, I have a love–hate relationship with snacks. Even though I'm a pediatric dietitian, it doesn't mean I'm immune to the struggles with snacking. Yes, I have kids who love junk food. Sometimes a little too much, thank you very much. I've had kids who want to snack when it's not time to snack. And, when they were younger, some of my kids would gladly skip a meal if it meant they could eat more snacks instead. Yes, there were days I hated snacks and was certain they'd derail all my efforts to raise a healthy eater.

But, as a pediatric dietitian, I also love how useful snacks can be to a child's health. They can close the gap on nutrients a child may not be getting at mealtimes. They can be a tool to help a child better regulate his appetite. And they can promote creativity, learning, and autonomy with eating. I know snacks can be—and should be—a joyful part of the eating experience during childhood.

I think it's fair to say you may feel the same way about snacks: You love them and you hate them.

So, how do we reconcile this love–hate relationship? How do we fall more in love with snacks and snacking? How do we cultivate a positive mentality around our kids' snacking and lose some annoyance? I believe it happens when we learn how to raise a *Smart Snacker*.

———

What is a *Smart Snacker*?

A *Smart Snacker* is a child who knows which combination of foods to choose for a snack, and how, when, and where to eat it to satisfy his appetite, cravings, and enjoyment. A *Smart Snacker* also knows that indulgent snacks are okay, and can balance them in the overall diet.

———

But before you learn to raise a *Smart Snacker*, you need to understand a few things: how we became so enamored with snacks in the first place, the impact of snacking on children's health, and why we rely on them.

How American Parents and Children Fell In (and Out of) Love with Snacking

Snacks came about in 1904, at the World's Fair in St. Louis. Then, the world was introduced to new foods including waffle cones for ice cream, Dr. Pepper (a soda), hot dogs, and cotton candy. Oreos were created in 1910 and by the roaring '20s and prohibition, the snacking industry was on a roll. World War II had a big impact on snacking, with a lull in innovation during rationing, but with a fierce resurgence later in the decade. M & M's and Cheetos were created during this decade and hence, our love of sweet treats and salty, savory snacks. The '50s brought the invention of fast-food restaurants. It's important to note that nutrition and obesity weren't concerns when these products were developed.

Then the '70s came and moms went to work outside of the home. The dawn of the *"I can bring home the bacon and fry it up in the pan"* began. But, in reality, moms had less time for cooking. The family meal waned and eating outside of the home gained traction. So did weight challenges in children. In fact, since the '70s, weight challenges, collectively called "childhood obesity," have increased three-fold, according to the Centers for Disease Control (CDC) (Centers for Disease Control, 2018). Of course, moms going back to work is only one factor. As our cultural values and norms have evolved, we've realized some unforeseen consequences.

In the '80s, and through the mid-'90s, the trend of eating outside of the home persisted. Fast food, take out, and pre-prepped, cooked-at-home meals have been the norm ever since; but recent studies show eating outside of the home has leveled off to about 28–35% percent of families in the 2000s (Smith, 2013).

From the invention of fast-food restaurants in the '50s to

100-calorie snack packs in the new millennium, snacking and snacks have evolved from simple, whole foods from the fridge to an industry cranking out a plethora of packaged, convenient concoctions.

Now we're in a tough place. We enjoy these products but also know their use may not always be healthy. Before we blame the snacking industry and its detrimental impact on health, let's acknowledge this: We've been asking for these products. We're a busy society. And we want to feel nourished and healthy. A quick, convenient snack helps us meet that yearning. We also value food variety and ethnic cuisines, so we reach for new, creative snacks on the market. We love convenience and want instant gratification, so we eat a bar instead of a meal.

In fact, our love of snacking is affecting our meal habits. According to a 2019 report by *Food Dive*, 59% of adults would rather snack than sit down for a meal (Devenyns, 2019).

But, as I stated earlier, we dislike snacks, as well. We loathe them because our intuition says they're taking over our kids' diets. And that doesn't feel right. We're irritated by snacks because our kid seems to have a preoccupation with them. And, yes, we may even feel a little resentful because eating them may provide greater enjoyment to our kids than the meals we labor over.

These feelings about snacks and snacking come from missing the key information we need to get snack foods right. It's good to want to teach your child healthy habits around snacking. But before we can do that, you need to appreciate the stronghold and role they play in children's daily eating and diet composition. Let's look at the hard data on children's snacking.

The Stats on Kids' Snacking

Snacks are prevalent in the diet of American kids. Snacking is a term that refers to two things: the eating habits around snack foods such as timing, frequency, and location, and the snack foods themselves, which can be nutritious or not.

Let's look at young kids first. In a 2017 study in *Maternal and Child Health*, researchers looked at the contribution of snacks to the overall dietary patterns of 2-to-5-year-old children (Shriver, 2017). They found:

- More than 25% of their daily calories came from snacks
- Snack foods contributed almost 40% of the added sugar in their diets
- Cookies and pastries contributed the most calories, sugar, and fat, followed by sugary beverages

In older kids, a large survey of US children aged 2–18 years showed they snack about four times each day (Health Affairs, 2010). Food Navigator, a news outlet for food and beverage innovation, found this to be true, showing that school-age kids were eating, on average, over four snacks per day. Teens? They were eating just under four a day. Some kids, however, were consuming up to ten snacks per day! (Watson, 2013)

When you put it all together, snacking serves up the equivalent of a fourth meal for kids. That's a hefty contribution of nutrition, so it makes perfect sense to pay attention to getting those nibbles right.

Speaking of snacks, what exactly are kids eating?

On average, kids reach for cookies, chips, and other treat foods most often, according to research studies and surveys. These add up to about 600 calories per day (168 more calories than what they consumed from snacks in the 1970s). Comparatively, children aged two to six years are showing the highest increase in snacking, consuming an extra 182 calories per day compared to their same age counterparts from the '70s.

And if you think the above doesn't apply to your child, think about the snacks eaten outside of your home. They're probably not apples and peanut butter, nor hummus and carrots.

There's another trend happening too. Like adults, kids are eating less at meals and more from snacks. The danger? Tipping the overall diet to an unbalanced place, especially if food choices reflect the research trends. So what does this mean for your child's health? Snacks and snacking habits can contribute to poor food choices and overeating, potentially leading to nutritional deficiencies and weight concerns.

Despite this gloomy outlook, there is good news.

Parents are trying to get snacks right. Thirty percent of parents are trying to establish healthy habits around snacking, and opt for healthier snacks for their kids, according to a 2015 report from Mintel, a marketing research firm (Topper, 2015). More good news: This book will help you do just that.

THE SNACK SEDUCTION IS REAL

Even though snacking can be part of a healthy diet, the statistics tell us we're victim to it. We can't deny the pull towards snacks and snacking. Why did we get so far off track with snacks?

We Are Busy, Busy, Busy

We are one busy bunch of parents. I know I'm busy. My friends are busy. And my clients are busy. Whether you're working in or out of the home, have outside commitments, or are managing online learning, after-school activities, music lessons, religious obligations, or other factors, it doesn't change this: You're likely facing one big time crunch.

When you have little time, you need quick food solutions. Enter packaged snacks, vending machines, and quick marts. Yes, they're convenient and efficient. But are they healthy? And do they encourage healthy eating habits?

The Snack Options Are Endless

The snack food market has exploded over the last five years, moving from a $3 billion industry to a $23 billion industry in 2018, according to an industry analysis report (Grand View Research, 2019). In part, the hectic lifestyles of families have propelled the snack market forward. From popcorn varieties to every type of granola bar you can imagine, food companies keep cranking out the variety of snack options, working to make them more convenient and more nutritious.

Snacking Opportunities Are Everywhere

Snacks are ubiquitous—they're everywhere. Of course, our homes showcase pantry and refrigerator snacks. And traditionally, our schools, after-school programs, churches, and sporting fields have offered the same. Parents have to account for additional snacking, both planned and unplanned.

Some Snacks Have Addictive Qualities

A 2013 article published in *The New York Times Magazine* detailed the path of addiction to junk food (Moss, 2013). Between fat, salt, and sweet flavors coupled with crunch, crispness, color, and appearance, ultra-processed snack foods may hook the palate.

Scientists create snacks with the "bliss point," or the point of sheer enjoyment and memorability, in mind. So if your child seems hooked on chips, crackers, and cookies, you're not dreaming. There's a planned, scientific approach to getting all humans to like ultra-processed snacks.

Kids Are Subject to the Shiny-Object Syndrome

Added to the addictive qualities of processed snack foods, you've got corporate America marketing their goods to your child. Just walk into a grocery store and look through her eyes. You'll see colorful boxes and characters, placed at eye-level on endcaps and at entryways, chock full of snack foods. TV commercials, online programs, and digital games tempt your child further. And they cause another dilemma for you: The pester factor. Kids beg for snack items, and parents often succumb.

Snacks Are a Comfortable Crutch

I'll never forget my high schooler's first final exams. A letter went out to the parents to inform them the school would provide snacks during exam week. I made some suggestions to the committee. Things like whole fruit, jerky, and mini bagels. The reply?

"Kids and teachers look forward to packaged cookies, chips, and candy."

We need to acknowledge that "snacks" may be permission to eat unhealthy foods, as this story describes. Yes, it's easy to get stuck in a routine with snacks and get caught up in a mindset of indulgence. What you grab for yourself can be a mindless endeavor. This goes for giving your child a snack too. We rely on the same snacks, day in and day out. While this is easy and requires little thinking, this is a crutch and it stifles food variety.

Let's Take Back the Snack!

We can take back the snack by learning to fall in love with snacks again. But not like before, where it was about the innovation and taste, then later moved to convenience. No, we fall in love with snacking when we master the skills needed to feed our kids healthfully without giving up food enjoyment.

One thing's for sure: Snacks aren't going away. The snacking industry is growing by leaps and bounds. While snacks can aid your child's growth and development, they can also hinder it. So it's up to you, *Smart Mom*, to make the right decisions for your child so you can raise a *Smart Snacker*.

I know it can feel as if you're fighting an uphill battle. In today's world, it's easier for your child to become a junk-food snacker than a *Smart Snacker*. Let's take back the snack. Let's put snacks to work *for* your child. I know you can do this when you're more knowledgeable about snacks, including what to serve, how to feed them, and how to navigate the challenges that come with them.

Why I Wrote This Book

I wrote *The Smart Mom's Guide to Healthy Snacking* to help you navigate one of the most challenging aspects of feeding and raising kids. There's no denying snacks are a central part of every child's diet. Parse out the daily routine of feeding kids, and you'll find you're making about 28,000 meals and snacks over your child's childhood (18 years). That's a lot of meals and snacks!

Snacks make up about 28% of a 2-to-5-year-old child's energy intake and 27% for older kids (Shriver, 2017). That's more than a quarter of what they eat in a day. It's critical to get this part of feeding right.

I also know that snacks and the habits of eating them are a

pain point. As I mentioned earlier, we love snacks and we hate them. I know if I can help you see snacks in a new light and give you some strategies and new ideas, you'll feel better about your child's eating. A game plan like this helps any parent feed better —and *feel* better!

The Smart Mom's Guide to Healthy Snacking helps you master snacks, including their timing, frequency, and nutritional composition. More importantly, this book will help you:

- Understand the role of snacks in your child's diet
- Identify how many and how frequently your child should be eating snacks
- Focus on nutrients that satisfy and help your child manage his appetite
- Plan healthy snacks using my simple step-by-step method
- Load up on creative, healthy snack ideas and ways to serve them
- Navigate tricky snacking situations such as constant complaints of hunger, overeating snacks, sneaking snacks, and snacking outside the home
- Get inspired by healthy snack combinations and simple recipes

How to Use This Book

In this book, you'll learn the general concepts around raising a *Smart Snacker* through the acronym "SNACK SMART."

SNACK SMART stands for:

S – **Snacking Intervals:** Set up a schedule and rhythm for feeding snacks.

N – **Nutrient-Rich Foods, Most of the Time**: Focus on nutrients in foods; balance sweets & treats.

A – **Amounts Matter**: Start with age-appropriate snack portions.

C – **Calories Count**: Fill up and satisfy your child with QC (quality calories).

K – **Keep It Contained**: Set boundaries to improve snacking.

S – **Simple & Easy**: Build your toolbox of healthy snack options.

M – **Monitor & Model Eating**: Parent in a way that encourages healthy habits.

A – **Appetite Awareness**: Support self-awareness of appetite and satisfaction.

R – **Responsive & Flexible:** Promote independence—let your child take the lead.

T – **Temperament & Development**: Understand what motivates your child.

I devote each chapter of this book to outlining each letter of the acronym, giving you the details and science behind what really matters so you can make the best decisions for your family. You'll be asked at the end of each chapter to put your knowledge into action so you can start reshaping your child's snacking habits right away.

The chapters are brief and to the point. I know from past feedback that this is practical for busy parents like you. Keep this book in the car to devour in the school pickup line, on your bedside table for a quick pre-sleep read, or take a 15-minute reading break before the kids arrive home from school. I promise, this will be a quick, digestible read, and one that you can put into practice right away. That's the goal, anyway.

As you read, you'll get snack ideas, creative food combinations, some homemade snack recipes, and kid-friendly ways to serve snacks. By the end of this book, my goal is to make you a *Smart Mom* (and your child a *Smart Snacker*) who routinely offers healthy snacks and promotes healthy snacking habits.

So, let's get started!

S N A C K S M A R T: S

S IS FOR STANDARD SNACKING INTERVALS

Alyssa's kids were free-range eaters. They breezed in and out of the kitchen, helping themselves to snacks. They'd quip, "Mom, I'm hungry!" and she'd reply, "OK, help yourself from the snack drawer."

The problem was, her kids were in the snack drawer several times a day.

"I thought letting my kids be independent in choosing their snacks was a good idea, but now I'm just feeling frustrated," she said. "I thought I was promoting their independence, but it's turned them into kids who've developed a bad habit of snacking too much."

Alyssa's frustration highlights what can happen when kids don't have a regular snacking schedule. For some kids, the independence associated with a snack drawer or even an "open" kitchen policy (we'll explore this concept later in the book) can be too much to handle.

While kids love this freedom, they don't know how to control it, or themselves. We need to help them.

Enter the first principle I'll cover: Letter "S" of the SNACK SMART acronym: *Standard Snacking Intervals*.

Before I set you up with a suggested schedule for snacking, you need to understand why snacking intervals are important, how they help your child, and why they support your child's growth and development.

Digestion 101

As I mentioned in the Introduction, digestion is a complex process, involving a number of different organs within the body (KidsHealth from Nemours). Hormones, enzymes, and other elements factor into this process too. Let's simplify this concept for now. We'll dive in deeper in Chapter Eight.

Think of the stomach as a balloon. It already contains some acidic juices. When we eat, it fills up and stretches to accommodate food. These juices start breaking down food into smaller pieces. As this is happening, food moves out of the stomach and into the intestines. Over two to three hours, most of the stomach contents will make the journey to the bowel.

If you eat a small amount of food, like a snack, the stomach will empty sooner. If you eat a meal, it will take longer to empty. Certain components of a meal, like fat, can slow down the process, keeping the contents in the stomach longer. Of course, other factors can speed up stomach emptying (think food poisoning, for example), or slow it down (not enough fiber).

As the stomach fills up, it fires a hormone to the brain called leptin. Leptin tells the brain and body it's full and need not eat any longer.

When the stomach is empty, the stomach signals the brain

telling it it's hungry. This signal is the hunger hormone called ghrelin (think *GHRRRR*elin for hunger).

These hormones regulate hunger and fullness and provide an internal message telling your child when to eat. When they eat frequently, such as every hour or two, they don't create enough time for the stomach to empty and signal hunger. In fact, this can interrupt those hormone cues altogether.

Alternatively, if kids eat in response to the triggers of hunger and fullness, you may see longer periods between eating sessions.

Imagine the power of teaching kids to eat in response to their appetite cues! We'll dig into more details around appetite in Chapter Eight, as it's an important concept for healthy snacking.

GROWTH AFFECTS THE TIMING OF SNACKS

As your child grows, his body and its organs get bigger. Stomach included. For example, an infant has a tiny tummy. Babies eat about every 1.5–2.5 hours in the first few months. If you've noticed, the early days of infancy are packed with frequent feedings—around twelve eating sessions a day. As the infant grows, his eating intervals stretch out to about every two to three hours by the end of the first year.

A toddler's tummy is small, too, but bigger than an infant's. When the tummy can hold more food, it can endure more time between eating sessions without spurring the appetite hormones. And so it goes. A child's belly can hold more food than a toddler's, and a teen's tummy can hold more than a child's. In fact, an adolescent's stomach can hold similar quantities as an adult's.

As the stomach grows and holds more food at once, the time to digest and empty the stomach (and thus trigger the hormone ghrelin) is longer. As a result, the intervals between eating occasions stretch out.

While some of this may seem obvious, parents aren't always changing the snacking intervals and schedule when they need to. For example, I've met many kids over the years who are eating three and four snacks each day. This is too many.

THE BENEFITS OF PREDICTABLE ROUTINES

Alyssa's kids didn't really have a snack routine. They could access snacks whenever they felt like it. This led to frequent eating, which interrupted their appetite cues. Free-for-all snacks set her kids up for unhealthy snacking habits and eating too much.

When kids have a routine with snacking (and eating meals), they are better supported in their ability to regulate their appetite. Their bodies acclimate to the routine of the schedule, enabling them to better interpret the appetite signals their body is sending. They're 'tuned in' to their appetite.

Alternatively, when kids can frequently snack throughout the day, they may fall out of sync with interpreting hunger and fullness. In fact, sensing those signals can be hard. Instead, they rely on external factors, such as boredom, or a learned habit like heading to the pantry on a TV commercial break, to cue their eating. We see this with Alyssa's kids. They'd developed a habit of mindlessly heading into the kitchen to eat and were out of touch with their appetite. This made them increasingly at risk of overeating.

A snacking schedule also separates eating from other activities. When it's time for a snack, your child puts down his toys, turns off the TV, or comes in for a break from outside. These carved-out eating times throughout the day set up a framework that helps your child regulate his appetite and eating. And we know this ability is part of the foundation of lifelong health.

While you don't have to be rigid about the timing of meals and snacks, a set schedule helps keep things predictable. Of course, you'll want to have some flexibility because life doesn't always operate on a rigid schedule, or as planned. You can allow some wiggle room around the timing of snacks if needed, but don't be willy-nilly, serving them at odd times or only when asked. This can make your child unsure and insecure.

If a child is insecure about snacks or eating, you may see it's affecting his eating behavior. Rapid eating, frequent questions about when and what food is being served, sneak eating, or even emotional responses like crying or tantrums may show the food routine is too unpredictable.

Kids like to know when they can expect to eat, and what will be served. A predictable routine helps them feel more secure. And this helps them stay in sync with their body's cues for eating.

STANDARD SNACKING INTERVALS BY AGE

Based on everything you've learned about setting standard snacking times, let's dive into a recommended snack schedule based on different ages (Shield, 2019). These are approximations. Each child ideally relies on hunger and fullness cues to guide whether he eats a snack, and how much is eaten.

. . .

Young Children (2–4 years)

Toddlers and young preschoolers eat up to three snacks per day to meet their nutritional needs for growth and development. These snacks can be real food or they might be a cup of milk, especially for young toddlers who still drink quite a bit of milk. Remember, the tiny tummies of younger children make it important to offer frequent eating opportunities.

Young children will eat a meal or a snack every two to three hours.

School-age Children (5–12 years)

Kids in school need about one to two snacks per day. Younger school-age kids (ages five and six years) may still get three snacks each day and need to transition down to two snacks per day. The timing of this will depend on what's happening with their growth.

Children aged six to nine years typically eat about two snacks per day. Older school-age kids, such as those aged nine through twelve years, will do well with one or two snacks per day, depending on their daily schedule and activity level. Active kids may need more.

The good news is, many schools allow time for a morning snack. Hopefully, this is nutritious. A child's second or only snack usually occurs after school.

School-aged children will eat every three to four hours.

Teens (13–18 years)

Teenagers are like adults. They can handle more food at a sitting and they can go longer between eating sessions. They do well with three meals and one snack each day, unless they are an athlete requiring more nutrition to accommodate athletic training, or are in a growth spurt and need additional calories and nutrients.

Like adults, teens eat every four to five hours.

———

How Many Snacks a Day?

Toddlers and Preschoolers: (2–4 years): 3 snacks per day

Young School-age Children (5–6 years): 2–3 snacks per day

School-age Children (7–12 years): 1–2 snacks per day

Teens (13–18 years): 1 snack per day

———

SAMPLE SNACKING SCHEDULE

For all kids, following a snacking schedule helps them meet their nutritional needs and avoid getting too hungry. Try to set a daily snacking schedule that stays consistent in your home. Of course, things can get busy, like when you have to make an extra trip to school and drop something off or pick up your child early. Your "ideal" schedule may be a bust. That's okay. You can be flexible in these situations. You may have a child who's feeling extra hungry sometimes. That's okay too. Offer a piece of fruit or other nutrient-rich option in this case.

On a typical day, here's what your child's snack schedule might look like:

For the Toddler

Mid-morning snack at 9:30 a.m.
Mid-afternoon snack at 2:30 p.m.
Bedtime snack at 7:00 p.m.

For the School-age Child

Mid-morning snack at 10:00 a.m.
Mid-afternoon snack at 3:00 p.m.

For the Teen

Mid-afternoon snack at 3:30 p.m.

NIBBLE ON THIS

As you can see, when we tie snacking times to the ebb and flow of normal digestion, we can help kids become more attuned to their appetite and get better at self-regulation. Setting up a predictable snack schedule can be your ally for keeping your child satisfied and nourished, while also supporting awareness of his hunger and fullness cues.

Alyssa got rid of the snack drawer and implemented regular snack times. The schedule became a routine and her kids got used to it, knowing when they could have snacks, and when they couldn't. It took some time to reverse some of their snacking habits, but Alyssa leaned on the predictability angle of her new routine, reinforcing when her kids could expect snack time.

Next, you'll learn about the second letter of SNACK SMART. "N" is for *Nutrient-Rich Foods, Most of the Time*. Get ready to explore the importance of nutrients in snack foods.

. . .

Take the Challenge!

Jot down the times you'd like to serve snacks to your child based on the intervals that make sense for his age and the number of snacks he needs for the day. Try to stick with this timing for the next two weeks.

2

SNACKSMART: N

N IS FOR NUTRIENT-RICH FOODS, MOST OF THE TIME

Janet's boys, Joey and Robbie, come home after school and head directly for the pantry. After a split-second scan of the contents (and a few "We have nothing to eat!" comments), they start their after-school snacking on crackers, cookies, popcorn, cheese, and chips.

They eat whatever they can get their hands on—and lots of it —before they move on to homework. Meanwhile, Janet makes suggestions like, "Why don't you have an apple?" Sometimes she shouts, "That's enough cookies!"

Janet wants her boys to eat healthy after-school snacks. They're growing, active, and impressionable. She knows what they eat is important to their health and well-being. But she's got too many sweets and treats in the house, and it draws her boys to them like a magnet.

"I buy what my boys like to eat, or what they request," Janet told me. "I know fruits and vegetables are healthy, but outside of that, I don't know what else to give them."

Janet needed a crash course in nutrition. She needed to understand that snacks can be an ally in meeting her boys' nutrient needs, and she needed to know her options. Specifically, where to find them in food.

In this chapter, I'm tackling the letter "N," the second letter in the acronym, SNACK SMART. "N" stands for *Nutrient-Rich Foods, Most Of The Time.*

The nutritional quality of snacks can make or break the daily diet. Healthy snacks contribute nutrients while unhealthy snacks can fall short. It's commonly known that when kids get the nutrients they need, they grow well and can maintain their health. That means fewer illnesses today, and better resistance to chronic disease tomorrow.

In this chapter, you'll learn about some of the most important nutrients for kids, where to find them in food, and how to fit snacks containing sugar and fat into a healthy snack plan.

Snacks Are Not Created Equally

There's a wide variety of snacks available. From natural, wholesome foods to ultra-processed ones, the plethora of choices range in their nutritional quality. Some are chock full of nutrition. Others are not.

Nutrient-rich is a term to describe food that contains an appreciable amount and a good variety of nutrients. For example, yogurt is a nutrient-rich food. It has anywhere from 8 to 15 grams of protein, about 300 mg of calcium, plus other nutrients like potassium, phosphorus, vitamin A, and more. There's a lot of nutrition in a single one-cup serving.

In contrast, nutrient-poor foods are foods that don't contain many nutrients, and if they do, they aren't in amounts that will really make a difference. Or, they may showcase nutrients that work against your child's health. For instance, chips are rich in salt and saturated fat, and candy contains a lot of sugar.

When your child eats a nutrient-rich food for a snack, it contributes positively to his overall daily intake. When she eats a nutrient-poor snack, she may tip her diet balance to an unhealthy place or crowd out the nutrients she really needs.

What Are the Nutrients Kids Need?

It may surprise you to learn that children need about 40 different nutrients each day to match their requirements for growth and development. Nutrients like protein, fat, and carbohydrate; calcium and vitamin D; and iron and fiber.

Let's spend some time delving into some of the most important nutrients for growing children so you can understand their role.

Protein, Fat, and Carbs

Protein, fat, and carbs are the major nutrients found in food. We call them *macronutrients*. They're often found alone or in combinations within foods. For example, you can find pure fat in oils and straight-up carbs in vegetables. It's pretty hard to find pure protein in food. It's usually packaged with the other macronutrients like milk or nuts. These macronutrients supply calories: protein and carbohydrate provide four calories per gram, and fat offers nine calories per gram.

Their sidekicks, the *micronutrients* (vitamins and minerals), are packaged alongside the macronutrients. They don't offer any calories. All macronutrients and micronutrients are important to growing children. While I will mostly focus on snack foods in this book, I want to give you a quick overview of why these nutrients are important to kids.

Protein

Protein is made up of amino acids that act together as building blocks for cells, organs, and muscles. Since growth is a dynamic building process, protein is needed every day. Protein is involved in building or repairing damaged tissues from the daily task of living and the natural muscle breakdown that happens with exercise. Protein is part of the hormones, enzymes, and other elements that make our bodies work. Children typically get enough protein from their diets without paying too much attention to it. That's the good news. The downside? Kids fall short in eating beans and fish, two of the best sources of protein.

———

Food Sources of Protein: Eggs, milk, yogurt, cheese, fish, beans, chicken, beef, lamb, pork, nuts, nut butters, seeds, quinoa

———

Fat

Fat is a concentrated energy source and provides essential fatty acids such as alpha-linolenic acid (ALA) and linoleic acid (LA), which the body cannot make itself. We must get these essential fatty acids from food. Fat is involved in brain development, especially in the first two years of life, which is why it's important for babies to get almost half of their calories from fat. Fat continues to be important for brain functioning throughout childhood. It helps the body absorb vitamins A, D, E and K, and helps kids feel full, or satiated, after eating.

Of course, there are different types of fat, some of which contribute to overall health, and some which deter it. In fact, there are four different types of fat: saturated fat, trans fat, polyunsaturated fat, and mono-unsaturated fat. Let's take it from the unhealthiest to the healthiest forms.

Saturated and trans fats are the bad boys in town. They are hard at room temperature, like a stick of butter. Saturated and trans fats increase the risk for heart disease and stroke because they raise bad cholesterol (LDL) levels. We can see the signs of elevated cholesterol in childhood, and fatty streaks and cholesterol deposits in blood vessels around the heart. These are early signs of heart disease.

Monounsaturated and polyunsaturated fats are the good guys. These fats are liquid at room temperature, like vegetable or olive oil. They provide those essential fatty acids we can't make ourselves and lower bad cholesterol levels, preventing heart disease and stroke.

The way to fight the bad boys is to replace the saturated and trans fats with the good guys, monounsaturated and polyunsaturated fats. For example, instead of using butter, use olive oil.

———

Food Sources of Saturated Fat: Butter, whole milk, fatty meats like salami or steak, hard cheese, heavy cream

Food Sources of Trans Fat: Donuts, packaged cookies, bakery-made cakes and pies, microwave popcorn, frozen pizza, fried foods, stick margarine

Food Sources of Monounsaturated Fat: Olive oil, nuts, avocado, canola oil

Food Sources of Polyunsaturated Fat: Salmon, walnuts, sunflower seeds, flax oil or seeds, safflower oil

_____

Carbohydrate

Last, carbohydrates often get a bad rap. Yet, they're found in most foods and are packaged with a lot of goodness such as fiber, B vitamins, and iron. In fact, you can find carbohydrates in grain foods like cereal, bread, and pasta, and in dairy foods, vegetables, and fruit. They are fully present in most food groups, so 'cutting carbs' can be really challenging for kids, removing many foods and nutrients from their diet. Most importantly, carbs are a primary source of energy for the growing child, making up about half of a child's total caloric requirement for growth and development.

But, as most things go, there are some dark sides to carbs too. For one, sugar is a carb. While sugar isn't to be feared, it falls into that nutrient-poor category I described earlier. Unfortunately, with kids, it can be abused. Too much sugar means fewer nutrients for your child, and possibly too many calories.

The bottom line? Your child needs a blend of carbs, protein, and fat in his diet. Snacks can provide healthy sources of each of these, adding to the quality of nutrition your child gets every day.

_____

Food Sources of Carbohydrate: Breads, bagel, crackers, cereals, pasta, rice, potato, broccoli, green beans, lettuce, apple, banana, pear, strawberries, dried fruit, milk, yogurt, chips, candy, cupcakes, ice cream

_____

Vitamins and Minerals

Vitamins and minerals are the workhorses of the functioning body. Collectively, they keep the metabolism (the inner engine of the body) humming along, supporting the organs and bones, and processing the food we eat into the health we experience as living human beings.

Vitamins
───────

Vitamins come in two forms: fat-soluble and water-soluble. Fat-soluble vitamins, such as vitamins A, D, E and K need fat for transportation and absorption. For example, studies show that vitamin D from whole milk is better absorbed than vitamin D found in skim milk. That's because there is more fat in whole milk than skim.

Fat-soluble vitamins are stored in our fat tissue. As such, if mega-doses of fat-soluble vitamins are consumed, toxicity can occur. Also, if there's a lot of fat tissue, fat-soluble vitamins can be "sequestered" there, or stuck, disabling the vitamin from circulating in the blood. For example, in children with obesity, studies show that vitamin D can become "stuck" in fat tissue and less available to their bones.

Water-soluble vitamins, such as vitamin B and C, are carried and absorbed in water-based fluids, which means you need not worry about other nutrients being present for absorption. However, since water-soluble vitamins are *not* stored in the body, it means sources of these vitamins should be eaten daily so the body gets what it needs.

For instance, vitamin C is a water-soluble vitamin. When a food source like an orange is eaten, the body soaks up vitamin C to the point of saturation. We urinate surplus vitamin C out. It's like watering a pot of flowers. Flowers soak up the water to a point of saturation. Once saturated, the pot drains the excess water out of the bottom. We process water-soluble vitamins the same way. We have to keep "feeding" water-soluble vitamins to our bodies daily.

Minerals

We find minerals in soil or water. They are absorbed by plants or eaten by animals, which is how they enter our food supply. Some minerals, like calcium, are needed in large amounts daily, while others, like iron, are trace minerals because they're needed in smaller amounts.

Some minerals found in food are calcium, phosphorus, magnesium, potassium, sodium, zinc, iron, copper, manganese, iodine, and fluoride.

SHORTFALL NUTRIENTS FOR KIDS

There's been an abundance of research in kids that tell us what kids eat, how much, and which nutrients are missing or in surplus in their diets. This information comes from independent research and population surveys. Nutrients in low supply are called shortfall nutrients. According to the food intake surveys and the Dietary Guidelines for Americans (DGA), the shortfall nutrients for kids are a mix of vitamins and minerals, including calcium, vitamin D, potassium, fiber, iron, zinc, and omega-3 fatty acids (Dietary Guidelines Advisory Committee, 2020).

While there are children who meet all their nutritional requirements through a healthful diet, the reality is many do not. Paying attention to the shortfall nutrients can go a long way to keeping your child healthy.

The helpful thing about nutrients is that many of them show

up together, as partners in food. It's like they're married. Take iron and zinc. Often, they are naturally packaged together in foods (example: beans and beef). The same goes for calcium and vitamin D. You'll find them together in milk and in some other dairy products. Fish offers vitamin E and omega-3 fatty acids.

This natural packaging makes it easier to track and ensure your child gets the key nutrients he needs. So, if you're wracking your brain and starting to get stressed out about 40 different nutrients to keep track of...don't. Remember this: If you find one key nutrient in food, you'll often find its partner. Paying attention to a small list of nutrients, especially the ones that are known to be "at risk," will allow you to keep track of the bigger picture.

But first, let's look at the shortfall nutrients so you can have a better understanding of what they do and why they're important. Keep them in mind as you plan the nutrient-rich snacks you offer to your child.

Calcium and Vitamin D

Calcium is found in our bones and teeth. In fact, it's said that ninety-nine percent of the calcium in the human body is located there. Our bodies cannot make calcium. We have to get it from our diet. We naturally lose calcium through our sweat, skin, hair, nails, urine and feces (poo).

Most children meet their calcium needs up to age four. After that, calcium is an under-consumed nutrient (U.S. Department of Agriculture, 2016). A third of teen girls don't meet their calcium needs.

The most familiar role of calcium is in making your child's bones hard and dense, which is called bone mineralization.

Calcium also aids in normal muscle contraction and helps the blood clot. It supports communication throughout the nervous system, sending messages from nerves to muscles.

As a key element in muscle contractions, the body tightly controls and regulates calcium in the blood. All muscles, including those of the heart, lungs, gut, legs, and arms, rely on sufficient levels of calcium in the bloodstream to contract normally. Maintaining calcium in the bloodstream is so important that the body will do everything it can to make sure blood calcium levels stay in a normal range. That means if the body isn't getting enough calcium in the diet, it will take calcium from its reservoir (the bones) to ensure normal blood calcium levels.

As mentioned, the body stores calcium in our bones. This is the calcium "bank." During childhood, we deposit calcium in bone, building up strength, hardness, and density. By the time your child is around 20 years old, he or she has completed the bone-building phase and has achieved what we call *peak bone mass*. This is the highest bone mass and density your child will achieve in his lifetime. Obviously, optimal calcium consumption throughout the first two decades of life promotes dense, hard bones in adulthood. Or a full bone bank account.

During the adult years, bone density stays steady as long as we consume adequate calcium. However, if there is inadequate calcium in the diet, the body makes a withdrawal from the bank (bones) to keep calcium in the blood at a steady level. This balancing act is ongoing: Eat enough calcium in the diet and the bank is flush; eat less than enough calcium in the diet, and we make a withdrawal of calcium from the bank. The goal is for children to eat enough calcium-rich foods every day so they build a large bank account. This is the best defense against osteoporosis and associated bone complications later in life.

Vitamin D is both an essential nutrient and a hormone. It's a strong partner nutrient to calcium, acting as a helper in bone mineralization. Vitamin D enables the body to deposit calcium into bones, making them harder and stronger.

Vitamin D also plays a role in keeping the immune system strong, improves mood, and seems to protect against certain cancers, respiratory illness, heart disease, neurodegenerative diseases, and both type 1 and type 2 diabetes (Office of Dietary Supplements, 2020).

Roughly half of toddlers and preschoolers meet their vitamin D requirement from food sources, and less than half of school-age kids do. It's worse for teens: Only 40% of teen boys and 25% of teen girls get enough vitamin D.

We can get vitamin D from food, but there are few naturally occurring sources. Most of the food sources of vitamin D, such as milk, orange juice, and eggs, are fortified with vitamin D. Even with these options, most kids fall short on getting enough of this important vitamin.

Another potential source of vitamin D is from the sun. When ultra-violet B (UVB) rays reach the skin, they activate the body's natural source of vitamin D. Depending upon where you live, and whether you use sunscreen when outside, sunshine may or may not be a sufficient way to get vitamin D.

If your child doesn't get enough vitamin D in his diet, from the sun, or from a vitamin D supplement, he is more likely to accumulate bone at a slower pace, may lose bone mass, have a lower bone density, and/or experience broken bones.

Iron and Zinc

Iron carries oxygen in the blood, and, as I like to say, it helps all the organs and cells breathe. Organs, cells, and muscles all need oxygen so they can operate properly and do the job of making the body function. Without adequate iron, symptoms of fatigue, weakness, paleness, poor circulation, and anemia occur.

Four percent of toddlers and preschoolers have an inadequate intake of iron. School-age children meet their iron requirement, but once the teen years hit, 20% of girls miss out on iron in the diet. Thankfully, teen boys do a good job of matching their needs.

In the young, developing child, iron is a critical component of brain development and aptitude. The brain needs iron to grow and develop normally, especially in those first five years of life. In fact, a 2017 paper suggests an absence of adequate iron early in life can be devastating to a child's intellectual abilities later on (Georgieff, 2017). Later, during the teenage growth spurt, and for girls during menstruation, iron is an "at-risk nutrient" because of blood expansion and iron losses through monthly periods, respectively. Iron requirements are higher for the teen than the child.

There are two types of iron: Heme-iron, which comes from animals; and non-heme iron, which comes from plants. Vitamin C can help the body better absorb non-heme iron foods. Whole and enriched refined grain products, such as cereal and bread, are major sources of non-heme iron in kids' diets.

In short, iron should be on your radar. It's found in meats, beans, fortified cereal, and some vegetables. Check the Appendix for a list of iron-rich foods.

Zinc is best known for its role in growth and development, and for the immune system. Zinc helps the immune system function properly, is involved in protein creation, wound healing, and basic cell division, including the creation of DNA. It's also required for the proper sense of taste and smell.

Most children get enough zinc in their diets, according to national surveys (U.S. Department of Agriculture, 2016). However, children from food-insecure homes (one in four children during the pandemic) may be at higher risk for inadequacy. Zinc deficiency is characterized by lack of growth in height, loss of appetite, and impaired immune function.

Red meat and poultry are wonderful sources of zinc. Other sources include beans, nuts, certain types of seafood (such as crab and lobster), whole grains, fortified breakfast cereals, and dairy products. The Appendix has a list of zinc foods and their zinc content.

Potassium and Fiber

Potassium assists the body's muscle contractions and helps regulate fluid and electrolyte balance, nerve functioning, and metabolism. High intakes of potassium may lower blood pressure, temper the effect of salt on blood pressure, and may minimize bone loss. Potassium also helps move nutrients into cells and waste products out of cells.

Most people get all the potassium they need from what they eat and drink, except for children (U.S. Department of Agriculture, 2016). Toddlers and preschoolers do well with meeting their potassium requirements; however, two-thirds of grade-schoolers and half of pre-teens don't meet the requirement. This is because of a lack of fruits and vegetables in their diets.

Sources of potassium in the diet include leafy greens, such as spinach and collards; fruit from vines, such as grapes and blackberries; root vegetables, such as carrots and potatoes; and citrus fruits, such as oranges and grapefruit.

Fiber plays a role in normal digestion and bowel movements. It is also linked to reducing heart disease, gastrointestinal troubles, and cancer. Studies have shown a link to weight control due to the fullness effect of fiber, and better blood sugar control when adequate amounts of fiber are consumed.

Forty percent of children under eight years don't get enough fiber in their diet, while about half of preteens do (U.S. Department of Agriculture (2016).

There are two types of fiber: Soluble and insoluble fiber. Soluble fiber absorbs water and turns into a mushy consistency like oatmeal, while insoluble fiber does not. It's more like a piece of celery in water. Most high-fiber foods contain both soluble and insoluble types.

Unfortunately, many children do not meet the recommended intake of fiber. If your child is constipated or has irregular bowel movements, check the fiber content of your child's diet. It may need to be increased.

We find dietary fiber in whole grains, fruits, vegetables, nuts, seeds, and beans. Your child will experience the positive benefits of a high-fiber diet when plenty of fluids, especially water, are present in the diet. For more fiber foods, go to the Appendix.

Vitamin E and Omega-3 DHA & EPA

Vitamin E is a fat-soluble vitamin with antioxidant abilities. An antioxidant protects the body from the damage of free radicals. An abundance of free radicals in the body contributes to heart disease and cancer. Vitamin E is also involved in immune functioning.

Nuts, seeds, and vegetable oils are some of the best sources of vitamin E.

National surveys suggest vitamin E is inadequate in the diets of Americans; however, it's also noted that it's hard to quantify the complete intake of vitamin E, especially from the use of oils in cooking (Office of Dietary Supplements, 2020). Following a low-fat diet places individuals at higher risk for inadequate intake of this vitamin. As a fat-soluble vitamin, excess intake, especially from supplements, can cause toxicity.

Docosahexaenoic Acid (DHA) is a fatty acid that makes up half of the fatty acids in the eye's retina. DHA is very important during the first 24 months of life and is found in breast milk and fortified in many infant formulas. It's needed for brain development, just like we need calcium for bone growth and health.

Eicosapentaenoic acid (EPA), DHA's partner, helps with blood flow and circulation in the brain.

Both DHA and EPA are essential. The body does not make them, so your child needs to get them from food or a supplement. Intake studies suggest a minimal amount of both DHA and EPA are consumed through food. Surveys suggest about 1% of US children use supplements containing fish oil, omega-3s, and/or DHA or EPA (Office of Dietary Supplements, 2020).

Throughout childhood, these fatty acids continue to play a role in heart health and brain functioning, especially problem solving, concentration, and memory. You can find a food list of these nutrients in the Appendix.

Where Can I Find These Nutrients In Food?

Now that you have a handle on the important nutrients for your child, where can you find them in food? Food groups, of course. Food groups are categories sorted by specific nutrients. There are five major food groups: Protein, Grains, Vegetables, Fruit, and Dairy. You can find more in-depth information about food groups at ChooseMyPlate (ChooseMyPlate.gov, 2020).

Fruit: This group includes all fruits, including fresh, frozen, canned, dried, and 100% juice. From berries to stone fruits (peaches and plums, for example), the fruit group highlights potassium, vitamin C, fiber, and other nutrients.

Vegetable: The vegetable group includes all vegetables, whether fresh, canned, dried, frozen, or 100% juice and breaks down this category of foods into subcategories: Red and orange vegetables, dark-green vegetables, starchy vegetables, beans and peas, and other vegetables. Subdividing vegetables further helps target nutrients and you'll find fiber, potassium, folate, vitamins A and C here. Here are some examples for each sub-category:

Red and Orange Vegetables: tomatoes, carrots, and sweet potato

Dark-green Vegetables: Romaine lettuce, spinach, and broccoli

Starchy Vegetables: Corn and potatoes

Beans and Peas (also part of the protein group): Pinto beans, black beans, black-eyed peas, kidney beans, and green peas

Other Vegetables: Onions, mushrooms, iceberg lettuce, green beans, and cauliflower

Protein: This food group includes a variety of meat sources like poultry, beef, and pork; eggs; seafood; beans and peas; nuts and nut butter; and soy products. The protein group highlights nutrients such as iron, zinc, vitamin B12 and other B vitamins, vitamin E, magnesium, and more.

Dairy: The dairy group includes milk, yogurt, cheese, and calcium-fortified soymilk. Other dairy products like cream cheese or butter are not part of the dairy group, but are in the fats and oils group. The dairy food group provides calcium, vitamin D (when fortified), potassium, phosphorus, and more. Of note, cheese and yogurt aren't typically fortified with vitamin D, but some brands are, so check the label.

Grains: This group includes any food made with wheat, rice, oats, barley, or other cereal grains. Bread, crackers, cereal, pasta, rice, grits, and tortillas are examples of foods from the grain food group. There are two types of grains: Whole Grains and Refined Grains. A whole grain has its grain kernel intact. An example is whole wheat bread. Refined grains are milled, removing the bran and germ. This process also removes fiber, B vitamins and iron. A good example of a refined grain is white bread.

We enrich many refined grains with certain B vitamins such as folic acid, niacin, thiamin, riboflavin, and iron, after processing. Fiber is not typically added back to a refined grain product; however, some grain foods are made with a mix of whole and refined grains and thus, would have some fiber content.

There are two more categories of food that I like to highlight, especially for kids: Fats and Oils and Sweets and Treats. These food categories will inevitably show up and contribute to your child's overall diet.

Fats and Oils: This category of food can be a significant calorie source in the foods your child eats. Although not an official food group, fats and oils provide nutrition. Solid fats are solid at room temperature and typically include saturated and trans fats, as explained earlier. Butter and shortening are easy examples, but you'll also find solid fats in coconut oil, chicken fat, and lard.

Oils are liquid at room temperature and are a source of monounsaturated and polyunsaturated fat. Examples are olive oil, canola oil, sunflower oil, vegetable oil, and corn oil. Some foods are naturally high in oils like nuts, olives, avocado, and some fish. These plant-based oils are heart healthy. Mayonnaise and salad dressing are mainly oils and you'll want to find types that are trans-fat free.

———

Wait... I Thought Coconut Oil Was Healthy!

Coconut oil has been the darling of celebrities and fad diets, like the ketogenic diet. Although it smells delicious and has some terrific cooking properties it's still a saturated fat. In fact, it's 100% fat, of which 80–90% is saturated. In 2020, the American Heart Association (AHA) reviewed seven controlled studies investigating the impact of coconut oil on blood cholesterol levels and found it raised LDL cholesterol (the bad cholesterol) in participants (Neelakantan, 2020). The AHA advises against using coconut oil, specifically, and saturated fats.

———

Sweets and Treats: For years, I've added sweets and treats to the food categories. I call them *Fun Foods*. They supply some nutrients, but are more likely to offer high amounts of fat and sugar, and thus, calories. Desserts such as cookies, cake, cupcakes, brownies, and candy fall into the Fun Food category. I also include here sugary beverages like soda and fried foods like French fries or chips. Like other food groups, identifying the foods and knowing what they offer allows you to balance them in your child's diet.

To summarize, food groups target the specific nutrients your child needs to grow and develop normally. Use them as the framework for planning snacks (and meals) so you're meeting your child's nutritional needs. Here's a summary of the nutrients you can expect from each food group:

———

Fruit: Vitamin C, fiber, potassium, folate

Vegetable: Vitamin A, vitamin C, fiber, potassium, folate

Protein: Iron, zinc, B vitamins (niacin, thiamin, riboflavin, and B6), vitamin E, magnesium

Dairy: Calcium, vitamin D, potassium, phosphorus, protein

Grain: Fiber, B vitamins (thiamin, riboflavin, niacin, and folate), iron, magnesium, and selenium

Fats and Oils: Vitamin E, DHA, EPA

Sweets and Treats: Sugar, fat

How Do I Use Food Groups to Plan a Nutrient-Rich Snack?

Making nutrient-rich snacks becomes a lot easier when you use the food groups. Of course, you can offer one food group, like a piece of fruit for a snack, but when you combine food groups you increase nutrients and potentially, your child's satisfaction. For example, instead of offering apple slices, give apple slices and peanut butter.

I call these *mini meals*. They comprise two or three food groups, instead of just one. Mini meals are more nutritious and they are more interesting and satisfying to children.

Mini Meal Snacks: Combine Food Groups to Create Nutritious Snacks

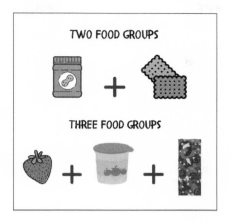

2 Food Groups

Fruit + Dairy = Strawberries and yogurt

Dairy + Vegetable = Cheese cubes and carrot sticks

Protein + Grain = Peanut butter and crackers

Dairy + Grain = Milk and cereal

Protein + Dairy = Turkey and cheese

3 Food Groups

Fruit + Dairy + Grain = Strawberry, yogurt, and granola parfait

Protein + Grain + Fruit = Almonds, dry cereal, and raisins trail mix

Protein + Vegetable + Grain = Hummus, cucumber, and pita bread

———

What about Sweets and Treat Foods?

Nutritious snacks will undoubtably improve the overall nutrition your child gets. But kids don't always want healthy snacks. Sometimes they want sweets and treats. Even though you do your best to make healthy options available, your child may get less than healthy options outside your jurisdiction. As one mom told to me, "Everywhere we go there is some kind of a sweet treat for my daughter to eat."

I know the lure of sweets, junk food, and other treats will tempt your child. There are reasons for this. For one, every child is born with a preference for sweet tastes. Amniotic fluid and breast milk are sweet. We imprint the familiar flavor of sweet early on. Second, the more sweet, salty, and fatty flavors a child experiences, the tendency is to like them more. And third, the food industry understands human tendencies and preferences. They orchestrate food products to capitalize on the addictive flavors of sweet, salt, and fat.

Sweets and treats, or *Fun Foods*, may be problematic in a child's diet if they are consumed regularly. Although some parents think their job is to ensure their children get NO *Fun Foods*, I'm here to tell you that doesn't work well in the long run. Plenty of research tells us that tightly controlling sweets and treats can backfire, leading some children to seek these 'forbidden' foods and overeat them.

Instead of being the food police around sweets and treats, there's another way. A way that helps kids learn to balance *Fun Foods* with nutrient-rich snack foods. Enter the 90–10 Rule. The 90–10 Rule emphasizes nutritious food groups, yet also includes a place for sweets and treats. It goes like this: Ninety percent of what your child eats comes from the food groups described above (fruit, vegetables, protein, dairy, grains, fats, and oils) and ten percent comes from sweets and treats, or *Fun Foods*. For most healthy kids, this ends up being one or two *Fun Foods*, on average, each day.

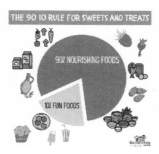

Let's use a real-life example to illustrate how this can play out. Sally knows they will offer her son donuts after church on Sunday, and cake and ice cream at the afternoon birthday party he's attending. She talks with her son about the *Fun Food* options that will come up for him, encouraging him to think about which *Fun Foods* he really wants. He must make a choice. He decides he will eat cake and ice cream at the party and skip the donuts at church.

Another example: Brent is playing baseball one afternoon, and he grabs a slushy drink. He passes on the bowl of ice cream later that night, remembering he chose his *Fun Food* earlier at the ballpark.

Of course, children will need help and guidance as they learn about *Fun Foods* and how to choose and balance them. It's important your child has a voice in determining which *Fun Foods* will be eaten and when they will be eaten. This means you are shifting a bit of the food decision-making over to your child in an area that may be most difficult for you and her to manage single-handedly.

Not only does the 90–10 Rule curb the unhealthy foods in your child's diet, it empowers her to make choices and self-regulate the amount of less-than-healthy foods she eats. If *you* choose the *Fun Foods* for your child, it will be less empowering and less effective in the long run. The goal here is to help your child pause and think through what she will eat during the day, and give her a tool to make nutritious choices, while thinking ahead and using her decision-making skills.

Nibble on This

Now you understand the importance of nutritious snacks in your child's overall snacking habits. While you don't have to be uber-healthy all the time, you want to create a balance of healthy and not-so-healthy snack foods. Even more powerful? Helping your child learn how to balance *Fun Foods* with nutritious snack foods. A balancing act that can last a lifetime!

Janet worked in more nutrient-rich snack foods and scaled back on buying so many chips and cookies. She also built in a rotation of snacking options at the ready when her boys came home from school. No more raiding the pantry or complaining about nothing to eat. Janet curtailed this by having nutritious snacks waiting for them when they got home.

In the next chapter, I'll explore the letter "A" in the acronym, SNACK SMART. The letter "A" stands for *Amounts Matter*. I hinted to this earlier when I described mini meals. You'll soon learn about the portion sizes for snacks, how to read a food label for serving sizes, and how to use nutrients to fill those tummies so they aren't hungry an hour later.

Take the Challenge!

Select two or three nutrients you want to focus on to

improve your child's diet. Create a list of foods that showcase those nutrients and work them into the snacks you offer during the week. For example, you may want to focus on calcium. Depending on your child's food preferences, perhaps you'll offer milk, yogurt and cheese; or cereal, soymilk, and almonds.

3

S N A C K S M A R T: A

A IS FOR AMOUNTS MATTER

J ack ate large portions, especially with snacks. He was
never full and always asking for more. The classic "bot-
tomless pit." Was he born this way? Or did he somehow
learn along the way to eat large amounts of food?

We'll talk about appetite later in this book, and how it can
influence how much we eat, but for now, let's explore the role of
portion sizes. It's trendy to live by the mantra 'less is more,' but
for food and eating, many Americans act on the idea that more is
better. Food manufacturers, restauranteurs, and fast-food establishments have caught on to this temptation, using sizeable
portions of food to lure folks in. All-you-can-eat buffets, "biggie"
gulps, and movie popcorn portions are just a few examples of
how portion sizes have gotten out of control. And let's be real.
It's hard not to be influenced by the mere sight of a large portion.

As a parent, you need to understand serving sizes and
portions so you're not overdoing it, nor underserving food to your
child. This makes it easier to model proper portions for your
child, so she absorbs this as the norm.

Welcome to the third letter in the acronym SNACK

SMART. "A" is for *Amounts Matter*. As you learned in the last chapter, the amount of food your child eats directly ties to the nutrients he's getting from food. The amount of food one eats is directly correlated to calories. The more you eat, the more calories you receive.

In this chapter, you'll get the starting point for portions based on your child's age, and learn how portion distortion and bigger portions increase the risk of overeating, even for children. So let's explore these concepts.

THE BASICS OF PORTION SIZE

How much food should your child eat? How do you know if you're over- or under-serving your child? Do servings change as your child grows? These are the questions about food amounts for kids that weigh on parents' minds.

First, let's get a few of the basics in our mind. A *serving size* is a standardized amount of food used to show a recommended amount to eat. For example, the food groups we explored in Chapter Two have recommended amounts, which we will delve into soon. The Nutrition Facts label, which you'll find on food products, details a serving size.

A *portion size* is the amount of food you eat. This may be more or less than a serving size.

Food portions for kids are smaller than they are for adults. No brainer, right? If you think about the size of a child compared to an adult, it makes sense that children would need smaller food portions. Their tummies are smaller and they need less food to fill them up. Yet, studies show that some parents serve their children the same amount of food they serve themselves. Obviously, this may be too much. As a result, children may learn that adult portions are the norm and end up overeating. By the time a child becomes a teenager, their portion sizes will approximate that of an adult.

Portion Distortion Is a Real Thing

Let's suppose you have a handle on serving sizes. You understand your toddler needs smaller amounts of food than you. You get that your child needs more food than your toddler. Great! But now you have to face the harsh reality of the food environment outside your home. Whether you're at the movies, out to eat, or trying to purchase a snack on the go, your child will be faced with opportunities to eat larger serving sizes. Serving sizes that may go far beyond his needs.

Just about everywhere you go, portion distortion exists. If we look back on the evolution of serving sizes, it's clear that they have grown over the decades. For instance, nearly fifty years ago, the size of the largest fast-food burger, fries, and soda was the same size as the smallest meal available today. That means a Happy Meal burger was the biggest burger you could get.

There are many examples of portion distortion. Take the movie theater. A small popcorn can easily meet the serving size for two people. Yet, it's not uncommon to be tempted by the value proposition of purchasing the bucket of popcorn and the biggest soda they offer...which could feed a small Boy Scout troop.

It's the same at fast-food establishments. Upgrade your order for more food. Or pay slightly more money and get the extra-large fries and drink. Pile your plate at the local all-you-can-eat buffet.

The worst thing about these large servings is that we

normalize them. We think a bucket of popcorn is the standard amount we *should* eat. We expect to get more value for our dollar, so of course, we'll take more food—often at the cost of ignoring our appetite and our health.

Snack foods aren't immune to portion distortion. It doesn't take much effort to find the extra-large granola bars, the inflated, single-serving bags of chips and crackers, or the packaged muffins that approximate the size of a newborn's head. Bagels, muffins, cookies, and trail mix are just some examples of how packaged snack serving sizes have grown over the years as well.

Fresh, whole foods are subject to this portion growth too. You can find three sizes of avocados and bananas. Even apples have gotten bigger!

THE TRAINING EFFECT OF LARGE PORTIONS

Understanding the serving sizes for children is an important concept to master. Portion distortion and larger serving sizes mean more calories (and yes, potentially more nutrients). If you're not aware of the proper serving sizes for kids, your child could get into trouble. Namely, getting excess calories—more than needed to grow well—which can cause extra, unhealthy weight gain.

Over time, the repeated offering of sizeable amounts of food may train your child to eat more than he or she needs. According to a review article published in 2010 by investigators from the Netherlands, the larger the portion of food served to adults, the more they ate (Steenhuis, 2010). It didn't matter whether they liked the taste of the food! Eating larger portion sizes persisted beyond the meal and participants did not cut back on calorie intake later on to compensate. In other words, they didn't down-regulate eating to compensate for fullness or the calories they consumed.

We also see this in children. Studies have shown when kids eat bigger portions, they aren't necessarily fuller, nor does it help them eat less food later on (Hetherington, 2018). And those *Fun Foods* we discussed in Chapter Two such as chips, cracker snacks, and desserts, may not satisfy your child's appetite. Your child may be hungry shortly afterward. The good news is those nutrient-rich food groups we discussed help your child's satisfaction and quell her hunger.

BEGIN WITH A STARTER PORTION

When it comes to food portions for kids, I like to teach an age-appropriate food portion to begin with (what I call a "starter portion") and then allow your child's appetite to guide how much he eats, including whether he has second helpings. When kids learn a reference point for a reasonable portion of food, they can visualize it, which can help them manage their eating.

I also deviate from the common term *portion control*. That feels restrictive and prescriptive to me and may lead to being too controlling with food. Measuring food intending to restrict or control food portions can become a negative feeding practice. I'll get into that in Chapter Seven. *Portion awareness*, on the other hand, can be a positive concept to teach your child. It's knowing what a reasonable amount of food is, and recognizing when the amount is too much. This awareness helps each of us make better decisions about how much food to eat.

To sum up, begin with a starter portion of food based on your child's age, and allow more or less food based on his or her appetite. For instance, eight-year-old Matt wanted a snack of cheese and crackers. His mom gave him five crackers and a cheese stick (one ounce). Matt gobbled it up and asked for more, stating he was still hungry. She gave him two more crackers and some water. Matt's sister, six-year-old Ava, got the same snack, but only ate four crackers and nearly all the cheese stick. She left the rest of the snack, stating she was full.

Portion Sizes for Children, by Age

The USDA *MyPlate* describes portion sizes for all Americans, except children aged 0-2 years (ChooseMyPlate.gov, 2020). While children need several portions of each food group daily, the reference point for how much to serve is your starting point. Remember, children should receive several servings and a variety of foods from each food group every day. Encourage your child to listen to his physical signs of hunger and fullness to gauge the amount he eats.

If five to seven crackers doesn't seem like enough for a snack, you're right. Remember, combinations of two or three food groups create a more robust, nutritious snack and a higher likelihood it will satisfy your child after eating it.

Below, I summarize the serving amounts for examples of food within each food group. For more examples, go to the USDA *MyPlate* website at https://www.choosemyplate.gov/.

A Portion for Young Children (2 to 3 years)

Protein: 1-2 Tablespoons of meat or beans; ¼ ounce of nuts; 1 to 2 teaspoons of nut butter; ½ to 1 egg

Grains: ¼ to ½ slice of bread or bagel; ½ cup cold cereal; ¼ to ½ cup cooked cereal; 2 to 3 crackers

Fruit: ½ to 1 small piece; 1/3 cup canned; ¼ cup dried; 1/3 cup juice

Vegetables: ½ small piece; ¼ to ½ cup leafy greens; 2 to 3 Tablespoons cooked; ¼ to 1/3 cup juice

Dairy: ½ to ¾ cup milk or yogurt; ½ ounce cheese

Oils: 1 teaspoon butter or oil; 1 to 2 teaspoons salad dressing or mayonnaise

A Portion for Children (4 to 6 years)

Protein: 1 to 2 Tablespoons of meat, 2 to 3 Tablespoons beans; ¼ to ½ ounce nuts; 2 to 3 teaspoons nut butter; 1 egg

Grains: 1 slice bread, ½ bagel; ½ to 1 cup cold cereal; ½ cup cooked cereal; 4 to 6 crackers

Fruit: ½ to 1 small piece; ½ cup canned or cooked; 2 Tablespoons dried; ½ cup juice

Vegetables: ½ to 1 small piece; ½ to 1 cup leafy greens; ¼ to ½ cup cooked; 1/3 to ½ cup juice

Dairy: ½ to 1 cup milk or yogurt; ¾ ounce cheese

Oils: 1 teaspoon butter or oil; ½ to 1 Tablespoon salad dressing or mayonnaise

A Portion for Children (7 to 9 years)

Protein: 2 ounces meat, ¼ cup beans; ½ ounce nuts; 1 Tablespoon nut butter; 1 egg

Grains: 1 slice bread, ½ bagel; 1 cup cold cereal; ½ cup cooked cereal; 5 to 7 crackers

Fruit: ½ to 1 cup or 1 medium piece; ½ to 1 cup canned or cooked; ¼ cup dried; ½ cup juice

Vegetables: ½ to 1 cup fresh; 1 cup leafy greens; ½ to 1 cup cooked; ½ cup juice

Dairy: ¾ to 1 cup milk or yogurt; 1 to 1 ½ ounces cheese

Oils: 1 teaspoon butter or oil; 1 Tablespoon salad dressing or mayonnaise

A Portion for Older Children (10 to 12 years)

Protein: 3 ounces meat, ¼ cup beans; ½ ounce nuts; 1 Tablespoon nut butter; 1 egg

Grains: 1 slice bread, ½ bagel; 1 cup cold cereal; ½ cup cooked cereal; 5 to 7 crackers

Fruit: 1 cup or 1 medium piece; 1 cup canned or cooked; ¼ cup dried; ½ cup juice

Vegetables: 1 cup fresh; 1 to 2 cups leafy greens; ½ to 1 cup cooked; ½ cup juice

Dairy: ¾ to 1 cup milk or yogurt; 1 ½ ounces cheese; 1/3 cup shredded

Oils: 1 teaspoon butter or oil; 1 to 2 Tablespoon salad dressing or mayonnaise

A Portion for Teens (13 to 18 years)

Protein: 3 ounces meat, ¼ cup beans; ½ ounce nuts; 1 Tablespoon nut butter; 1 egg

Grains: 1 slice bread, ½ bagel; 1 cup cold cereal; ½ cup cooked cereal; 5 to 7 crackers

Fruit: 1 cup or 1 medium piece; 1 cup canned or cooked; ¼ cup dried; ½ cup juice

Vegetables: 1 cup fresh; 1 to 2 cups leafy greens; ½ to 1 cup cooked; ½ cup juice

Dairy: 1 cup milk or yogurt; 1 ½ ounces cheese; 1/3 cup shredded

Oils: 1 teaspoon butter or oil; 1 to 2 Tablespoon salad dressing or mayonnaise

USE COMMON HOUSEHOLD MEASURES TO ESTIMATE SERVING SIZES

It's not always possible to measure food, or even desirable. Instead, you can use common household measures to approximate a starter portion of food. These give you an "eyeball" for food portions.

————

Common Household Measures

A deck of cards for 3 ounces of meat or fish

Three dice for 1 ½ ounces of cheese

A lightbulb for ½ cup of rice or pasta

A baseball for a cup or medium piece of fruit or vegetables, a cup of milk, or a cup of breakfast cereal

A poker chip for a Tablespoon of oils, salad dressings, and other fats

A hockey puck for a small biscuit or muffin

A CD for a serving size of a waffle or pancake

————

Another way to keep tabs on child-size portions is to downsize the plates you use for snacks and meals. For example, salad plates are much smaller than dinner plates and more reasonable for young children at dinnertime. I didn't graduate my own kids to large dinner plates until they were pre-teens. You can use a saucer, which is even smaller for snack time. Using a saucer or a salad plate makes the plate look "full" while keeping portion sizes to more age-appropriate amounts.

Creative ideas like bento boxes and condiment cups in measured sizes can also be a fun and creative way to serve kids appropriate portions of snack foods.

THE NUTRITION FACTS LABEL AND SERVING SIZES

You've probably looked at foods in the grocery store, turned over the package and noticed the Nutrition Facts Label. Maybe you use this tool already, or maybe you're confused by the information you see. Let's take a quick tour!

The Nutrition Facts Label is required by the Food and Drug Administration (FDA) on every food package. It's meant to help you understand the serving size and the nutrition you'll find within the food. Whether you want to know how many calories are present in a product, or are looking to moderate specific nutrients like saturated fat or sugar, the Nutrition Facts Label is an excellent source for this information.

On every package, you'll find the serving size and the number of servings in the package. For example, in a box of cereal, you may find the serving size to be 1 cup with 20 servings in the box. This serving size represents the amount of food people will typically eat. It's not a recommendation for how much you *should* eat.

They base all the nutrients listed on the label on the stated serving size. So, for our example of a cup of cereal, you may get 120 calories, 3 grams of protein, 1 gram of fat, 25 grams of carbohydrate, 4 grams of fiber, and 13 grams of added sugar. If your child eats two servings of cereal (or 2 cups), she'll get 240 calories, 6 grams of protein, 2 grams of fat, and so on.

The nutrients listed on the Nutrition Facts Label helps you watch out for unhelpful nutrients in your child's diet, like added sugar and saturated fat. It also helps you target nutrients we want children to eat, such as fiber, protein, and certain micronutrients like calcium, iron, and vitamin D.

Other micronutrients provided within a food product are listed as a percentage of what we need in the daily diet. It states this as a percent Daily Value, or % *DV*. The % DV helps you determine whether a product has a high or low amount of a certain nutrient in it. A 5% DV or lower is a low amount of that nutrient in the food product, while a 20% DV or higher is a high amount of the nutrient. For example, let's say our cereal example has 2% DV of iron and 30% DV of calcium. It would be considered a poor source of iron and a good source of calcium. While the % DV doesn't give you the exact amounts of nutrients within the product, stating it as a percentage of what your child needs daily allows you to determine good and low sources of specific nutrients. For more on understanding the Nutrition Facts Label, go to www.fda.gov (Food & Drug Administration, 2020).

NIBBLE ON THIS

Food amounts do matter in our overall eating patterns, weight, and health. Use the portion guide to target starter portions and the Nutrition Facts Label to guide your choices in packaged food. Let me be clear: I don't want you to restrict food to a certain portion, nor do I want you to disregard portion distortion. These are two potential extremes: too little food and too much.

Like Mama Bear in the *Three Little Bears*, I want you to get it "just right."

Jack's mom used starter portions for Jack's snacks. Instead of anticipating how much he'd eat in a sitting, she started with a reasonable amount of food and assured him he could have more if he was still hungry. The other thing she did was offer more than one food item for a snack, opting for a mini meal that was more filling. You can also do this with your own child by using starter portions and serving sizes, and allowing your child's appetite to guide the rest of her eating.

In Chapter Four, we'll run through the next letter in the acronym SNACK SMART. The letter "C" stands for *Calories Count*. While this topic can drum up visions of calorie counting and food restriction, my goal with this chapter is to help you not only understand calories, but encourage you to increase the *quality* of them so they strategically help your child be satisfied after eating. We'll do this through exploring the caloric contribution of snacks, including low-calorie snacks, added sugar in snacks, and key nutrients that encourage fullness.

Take the Challenge!

Practice using starter portions when you offer your child a snack. Use measuring tools or refer to the Nutrition Facts Label to guide you. Soon, you'll be able to estimate starter portions on your own!

4

S N A C K S M A R T: C

C IS FOR CALORIES COUNT

M aggie didn't have a good understanding of what she should offer for snack time. She struggled with making snack decisions, especially at the end of the school day. "Should I let her have a cookie?" she wondered. "No, that's too indulgent. I'll offer apple slices instead," she'd rationalize. But then her daughter would complain, whining that she wanted something else. They'd end up arguing about food, something Maggie didn't want to do.

When 100-calorie snack packs came out, they relieved Maggie. These little sweet and savory snack packs seemed to be the answer. Not only were they conveniently packaged in the right amounts, Maggie could find the cookies her daughter liked. Snack packs gave Maggie a sense of freedom. She didn't have to worry or fight with her daughter.

But that feeling was short-lived. Maggie noticed her daughter was eating several snack packs a day. She wasn't satisfied and complained she was still hungry. Maggie's worry about what and how much her daughter was snacking on returned.

Packaged snacks like 100-calorie snack packs, which are

portion and calorie controlled, may lure you in to thinking they solve your snack conundrum. They don't. Sweet treats aren't great for snack time, either. The biggest problem with these types of snacks is they may not satisfy your child's hunger, which means some kids will be back for more. If you're a superfan of snack packs, or serve up sweets at snack time, don't worry; there's a strategy to offer them so your child is satisfied and not begging for more.

In this chapter, I'm touching on calories, but I'm coming at them from a quality standpoint. I want you to understand the quality of calories from 100-calorie snack packs and sugary snacks versus those that include key nutrients that fill your child up and make those snack calories work for her. The big question I'll address: How can you ensure snacks contain the nutrients that make your child feel full and not ask for more before the next meal? And, of course, I'll offer you strategies, should you find that a snack pack or sweet is the only answer for your immediate situation.

CALORIE QUALITY: WHY ALL CALORIES ARE NOT EQUAL

I often hear "a calorie is a calorie." That's true, and it's not true. A calorie from cane sugar offers the same energy as a calorie from protein, but there are many more nutrients in a calorie from protein than cane sugar. A calorie from protein affects blood sugar, fullness, and brain activity differently than a calorie from a simple carbohydrate like sugar. In a nutshell, calories from different foods, and even nutrients, are not the same.

So what does that mean for your child's snacking habits? Nutrient-rich calories are more likely to have a positive impact on your child's overall nutritional status, weight, and feeling of well-being. Empty calories may have the opposite effect. We see this in studies of adults, like this 2011 *New England Journal of Medicine* study, which looked at 120,000 healthy women and men and their weight status over 20 years (Mozaffarian, 2011). The participants that consumed processed foods higher in starches, refined grains, fats, and sugars such as potato chips, fried potatoes, sugar-sweetened beverages, and both processed and unprocessed red meats, experienced more weight gain than those who routinely ate vegetables, whole grains, fruits, nuts, and yogurt.

THE QUALITY CALORIE (QC) CONCEPT

As with many things in nutrition, the nuances matter. With calories, quality counts. Foods with similar calories can be quite different in terms of the nutrition they provide. For example, one hundred calories from a handful of nuts will look very different from a handful of candy, nutritionally. A two-hundred-calorie snack of cheese, whole grain crackers, and fruit makes Goldfish crackers look weak from a nutrition standpoint.

The British Nutrition Foundation calls this idea the Quality Calorie (QC) Concept (British Nutrition Foundation, 2020). They focus on choosing wholesome, nutrient-rich foods so individuals are more likely to meet their nutritional requirements. They downplay foods with limited nutrients and/or nutrients associated with health risk, like sugar and saturated fat. The QC concept emphasizes the quality of foods eaten matters more than the number of calories consumed.

THE POWER OF PROTEIN, FIBER, AND FAT

. . .

Have you ever had a plate of eggs for breakfast and felt full well past lunchtime? Or ate a donut and felt hungry just an hour or two later? It isn't necessarily that eggs are particularly filling themselves, or that donuts cause more hunger. What makes eggs more filling and donuts less so boils down to their nutrient content, or whether they contain the nutrients of protein, fiber, or fat.

Studies suggest these nutrients encourage fullness, which can cause satisfaction and a desire to stop eating. The presence of one or a combination of these nutrients in a snack also keeps blood sugar evenly regulated, which may curtail food cravings. In a 2015 review study in *Trends in Food Science & Technology*, authors recognized that two foods of the same calorie content may have different effects on fullness because of their macronutrients (Chambers, 2015). Specifically, they outlined a hierarchy of satiating nutrients: Protein is the most filling, followed by carbohydrate, and then fat.

It's important to note that satiation, or the feeling of fullness, and satisfaction after eating are complicated responses to food. They span not only the nutrients present but also the perceptions and anticipation of eating, something we'll explore further in Chapter Eight. However, when we look particularly at the nutrient content of food and its impact on fullness, protein, fat, and fiber have plenty of research behind them.

How does protein affect fullness? Studies suggest there is an increase in thermogenesis, or the number of calories burned after eating, especially when animal-based proteins such as meat, eggs, or milk are eaten. We may interpret this increase in body temperature as satiety, according to a 2004 paper in *Nutrition and Metabolism* (Westerterp, 2004). Eating a protein-rich meal may also increase the release of gut hormones that tell us we've had enough to eat, potentially inhibiting appetite and causing a feeling of fullness, according to a 2017 study in the *British Journal of Nutrition* (Arguin, 2017).

Fiber, the source of carbohydrate most studies focus on, is more complex in its impact on satiety. Depending on the fiber, soluble or insoluble, and its ability to bulk up food, add viscosity (thickens a food product) or gel in the stomach, the overall effect is a feeling of fullness. Additionally, fiber-rich foods lead to stomach distention, a slowing of digestion, and encourages the release of hormones indicating fullness.

The satisfaction factor of fat is less clear. Studies have shown that when people can eat fat without restriction, they overeat. And despite more food consumption, an increase in energy intake does not equal satiety. However, the above 2017 *British Journal of Nutrition* study showed the power of a "satiating diet," one that is not restrictive of calories, but promotes the nutrients protein, fiber, and fat within food choices. Adult men who followed the "satiating diet" experienced weight loss, decreased percentage of fat mass, good adherence to the eating plan, and good satiety awareness.

The bottom line? The combination of protein, fiber, and fat can have a powerful effect on promoting fullness, which can be a useful tool when planning snacks for your child.

THE FLIP SIDE: 100-CALORIE SNACKS & SUGARY SNACKS UNDERMINE FULLNESS

Some parents are like Maggie, believing low-calorie snacks are a solution for your hungry child or for the child who likes to eat a lot of snacks. After all, when kids come home from school, they can be pretty hungry and want to dive in. If you're concerned about how much your child eats, or his weight, the inclination to limit calories or "healthify" them may be tempting. But as you learned above, this may be counterproductive.

Low-calorie snacks, particularly those 100-calorie snack packs, are often low in protein, and may have a higher sugar or refined carbohydrate content. Not exactly the stuff that will help your child get to the next mealtime. In a 2019 study from the *International Journal of Obesity*, researchers looked at the impact of pre-packaged snack items on children's and adults' eating patterns (Kerr, 2019). Children who were offered a higher number of snacks and more snack options ate considerably more calories and slightly more food quantity. Changing the package size didn't change the amount a child consumed. Pre-packaged snack packs didn't limit snacking, it increased it.

In my own experience of counseling children around snacking, I've noticed that few children are full and satisfied after consuming one pre-packaged snack, especially ones that limit calories. When kids eat, and are left feeling hungry, they ask for other snacks or more food to fill their bellies. Snacking can turn into a scavenger hunt for more food to feel satisfied, or full. The result? Poor snacking choices and overeating.

Sweet Treats Aren't Satisfying Either

Children eat a significant amount of added sugar in their diets, and most of it is served up at snack time. But sugary snacks have the same fate as low-calorie snack packs. According to the Center for Disease Control (CDC), kids are eating too much added sugar.

A 2018 study looking at the consumption patterns of added sugar in youth from 2005 to 2008 found that 2- to 5-year-olds were getting about 200 calories from added sugar per day (Bailey, 2018). Six- to eleven-year-olds were eating about 300–350 calories from added sugar each day, and twelve- to eighteen-year-olds were averaging 300–450 calories. Boys ate more sweets than girls, the sweets consumed were largely from food rather than drinks, and they were mostly consumed at home.

The American Heart Association (AHA) recommends that children's added sugar intake should be limited to **6 teaspoons per day**, or 96 calories per day from added sugar (American Heart Association, 2016). It's easy to see children are well over that limit. Prudently, they advise children under two years should skip added sugar altogether, according to the 2020 Dietary Guidelines for Americans (Dietary Guidelines Advisory Committee, 2020).

––––––

What Is Added Sugar?

Added sugar is the refined sugar added to foods during processing. It's different from naturally occurring sugar in food like fructose in fruit, or lactose in milk. The sugar found in candy, cookies, and cakes are obvious sweets and they contain added sugar. Examples of added sugar are cane sugar, agave, honey, maple syrup, and high fructose corn syrup.

Other foods have hidden sources of added sugar. They're not obvious or necessarily dessert foods. For example, cereal, spaghetti sauce, and yogurt contain added sugar.

––––––

Dessert foods full of sugar and fat do little to satisfy the appetite of a growing child. Sure, they taste great. The immediate boost to blood sugar may make a child feel great too, for a little while. But the rise and fall of blood sugar after eating sweets can make a child feel hungry and tired soon after. What happens next? They're asking for more food, whining, or being difficult.

How to Make Sweet Treats and Low-Cal Packaged Snacks Work

I don't blame you if you're reluctant to nix the low-calorie snack packs or the occasional sweet treat. They're convenient and pleasing. However, there is a way to use them to your child's advantage, making them more filling and satisfying. For one, never let them stand alone. Pair them with other healthy foods, such as a glass of milk (or milk substitute) or a piece of fruit. For example, if you're offering a cookie snack pack, pair it with a glass of milk. If you're serving a cracker or other grain-based snack pack, add fruit or cheese.

The same approach works for sugary snacks too. Pair them with a nutritious food to improve fullness and satisfaction. Here are some examples: Cookies and milk, candy and a whole grain mini bagel with nut butter, or a cupcake with fruit.

Nibble on This

One of the smartest things you can do is focus on the quality of calories you provide your child at snack time. Nutrients like protein, fiber, and fat are your ally in the quest to help your child eat healthy snacks and develop healthy snacking habits. After all, a child who is unsatisfied will want to feel satisfied, and that may mean seeking more snacks.

Maggie figured out a strategy for using snack packs, especially when she and her kids were on the go. She paired them with a nutritious food, like yogurt or a piece of fruit. She also included a sweet snack during the week, like cookies and milk, so her daughter got the cookies she loved, along with a nutrient-rich beverage. These work-arounds allowed Maggie to make the most of the convenience of snack packs without setting her child up for more snacking or letting them deter the overall nutrition quality of snack time.

While I've spent a bit of time on the nutritional quality of the foods at snack time, next I'm diving into boundaries, especially *where* kids eat snacks. In Chapter Five, I'll explore letter "K" of the SNACK SMART acronym, which stands for *Keep it Centralized*. You'll learn how to use boundaries to set up a healthy snacking environment at home, how to manage outside-the-home snacking, and tips for reducing sneak snacking. My goal is to help you use boundaries to teach your child healthy snack habits so they're transferable when she is out in the world on her own.

Take the Challenge!

Focus on adding a source of protein, fiber, or fat to your child's snacks this week and note her satisfaction level. Does she seem hungry or satisfied after eating? Experiment with different food sources and combinations to see which nutrients are most filling.

SNACKSMART: K

K IS FOR KEEP IT CONTAINED

J anine knew she was part of the reason her kids were out of control with snacking. In and out of the kitchen all day, they were constantly scavenging for something to eat. When she told them "no," they whined, acted out, and caused a scene. Admittedly, she hated to say no. It made her feel mean and unloving. It was easier to let her kids get what they wanted from the kitchen. But now things were completely out of control. Not only were Janine's kids eating too many snacks, they were essentially learning poor snacking habits that would become problematic to their health later on.

The statistics tell us that children are snacking way too much. Part of the reason for this is the lack of routine and limits parents have around eating, but especially around snacking. Unfortunately, I've seen parents who have a hard time saying no, or are uncomfortable with the fallout that ensues. I get it. No parent wants to be a "meanie." Yet, saying no, having limits around snacking, and following through with consequences are the cornerstones of parenting with regard to food and eating. In fact, they're the foundation of good parenting in any realm.

In this chapter, I'm diving into boundaries, or how to keep snacks contained as I explore the letter "K" in SNACK SMART. "K" stands for *Keep it Contained*. Setting boundaries will help you keep control of snacks and snacking and teach your child how to manage himself when you're not around. Without boundaries, you'll have a free-for-all in the kitchen, which may lead to unhealthy food choices and poor snacking habits. The limits you set around snacking will serve your child in and outside of your home. So, let's get started.

THE LOWDOWN ON FOOD BOUNDARIES

A boundary is *something that shows or fixes a limit or extent,* according to Merriam-Webster.

It can be concrete like the property line around a home, or abstract like the moral limit around stealing another's property, or lying. Food boundaries are the limits set around eating, including when your child eats, what he eats, and where. As your child's parent, you are the boundary setter.

Boundaries are very much part of our daily life. Think about the rules of the road, the rules in school, and the moral rules we've learned along the road of life. Without these boundaries there would be chaos. Car crashes and attendance problems in school are just some potential outcomes when rules are missing.

Rules around food and eating prevent chaotic eating and help support children in learning self-regulation with their eating. For example, eating food only in the kitchen contains food in one location, preventing less mess in other areas of the home. It also helps train children with good eating habits. Research tells us that eating in the car, in front of the TV, and in a bedroom encourages mindless eating. This may lead to overeating. These small limits can have great impact on building healthy eating habits.

———

What Is Mindless Eating?

Mindless eating is a lack of awareness of the food you're eating, including what you're eating, how much you're eating, and the sense of satisfaction or fullness when you're done eating. Outside influences may trigger it, such as a distraction, an emotion, or a habit. Eating mindlessly may become established in childhood. The opposite of mindless eating is *mindful eating*, or being present in the moment of eating with purposeful attention to the foods eaten, including the quantity, and the level of satisfaction or fullness after eating, which informs when to stop. Research suggests those who eat mindfully are better at enjoying the eating experience, eat less, and select foods that promote health benefits (Nelson, 2017).

———

How Boundaries May Help Improve Snacking Habits

Boundaries are powerful and they're one of my favorite areas to focus on with families, especially for snacking. Reinforcing limits around food access can help your child regulate his eating. In a 2017 review study in the *International Journal of Behavior, Nutrition and Physical Activity*, researchers concluded using rules and limits were effective in preventing unhealthy eating in children age seven and over. For kids age six and under, verbal praise that promoted healthy eating, like "Good job picking out a red fruit for your snack!" was more effective (Yee, 2017).

The example of Janine's kids highlights this research. They were eating all the time, mostly because they could. Janine wasn't saying "no," nor did she have a structure to back up her "no" in place. Her kids took advantage of this. When food limits are missing, kids don't have a stop gap. And if they're out of sync with their appetite signals, they may overeat. Overeating may create a sense of needing to eat more food to get the same sensation of fullness. This may further reinforce overeating.

Yet, putting boundaries in place can establish a rhythm and routine with eating, supporting (or re-establishing) the natural ability to self-regulate eating. Even better? The limits around food can transfer outside of your home, helping your child better navigate the world of food and the opportunities for eating when you're not around.

EASY BOUNDARIES TO IMPLEMENT

Boundaries can be as simple as the word "No," or "Not today," or more complex like the 90–10 Rule I explained earlier in Chapter Two. You've already learned about one boundary in Chapter One of the book: *Standard Snacking Intervals*. The simplicity of a set time for snacks is a key limit, or boundary, to healthy snacking. It sets the tone for when snacking happens and implies it won't happen otherwise. The following are some additional boundaries you can implement around snacking:

The Kitchen Is Closed

You can use the phrase 'The kitchen is closed,' to tell your child when it's okay to snack and when it's not. This boundary reinforces your designated snack times. When the kitchen is closed, it means it's off limits right now. For example, your kitchen may be open at 3:00 p.m. for snacks. After snack time is over, the kitchen is closed. Here are some other benefits of using 'the kitchen is closed' boundary:

- It allows time between eating sessions so that children can build up an appetite for meals
- It makes snack time predictable (as long as you're doing your part)
- Closing the kitchen supports a predictable rhythm of daily meals and snacks
- It diverts your child to other activities that have nothing to do with food or eating

Conversely, if your kitchen is always open and your child can get snacks whenever he wants to, then it will be hard to be your best at parenting your child around snacks. Snacking will be harder to monitor because you cannot accurately track your child's food consumption. Free-for-all access to food means your child is more likely to graze, snack frequently, and perhaps overeat.

The key to making 'the kitchen is closed' boundary work is making sure you have regular times when your kitchen is open. For example, "The kitchen is open for breakfast (or for lunch, snacks, etc.) at [xyz] time." Then, when your child comes to you an hour after eating breakfast, wanting something else to eat, you can say "the kitchen is closed right now," and set a clear boundary. If this is initially upsetting to your child, assure him that another meal or snack will be available soon. The kitchen is closed is a useful phrase when you've done a good job at providing meals and snacks on a predictable schedule throughout the day.

Sample Language: "Snack time is over and the kitchen is

closed. We'll open back up at lunchtime, which is at noon, or 12:00 p.m. Let me show you what twelve o'clock looks like (on the clock)."

Ask Before You Take

I learned the rule 'ask before you take' when I was a kid. And I carried on this boundary with my own children. 'Ask before you take' applies to a lot of things in life: borrowing clothes, a toy, or a coveted item. And yes, even food and eating. A simple, "You must ask me first," keeps you in charge of snacks and better able to monitor what and how much your child is eating. After all, the result of not having your child ask first is unregulated snacking. As a nutritional gatekeeper, you can use this boundary to allow or disallow sweets and treats or prevent overeating. Equally important, when your child follows this rule, you'll have a better sense of your child's daily snacking patterns.

Sample Language: "I see you're in the pantry. Are you hungry? If so, you need to ask me first before helping yourself. Let's figure this out together."

No Food Outside of the Kitchen

Establishing a regular place like the kitchen where your child gathers for snacks is key to helping her understand exactly where she needs to show up to eat. Of course, life isn't always predictable and you may find an occasional snack may be eaten in the car on the way to a game or school event. That's ok! There will always be circumstances that require you to change the usual snack routine; however, it's important to have a regular location for snacking in place. When an exception happens, let your child know it's an exception to the rule, not the norm.

Younger children should be trained to sit for snacks, rather than roaming throughout the house with a baggie of crackers in hand. Walking around while eating is an unhealthy habit that may disengage your child from the sensation of fullness.

Sample Language: "Sweetie, you know our rule is to eat snacks in the kitchen. Come on back and sit at the table."

Or: "We sit at the table for snacks. We'll play some more after snack time is over."

Always Eat a Nutritious Food with a Sweet Food
_____

It seems there's always an option for sweets and treats. They seem to pop up everywhere! Another boundary that helps your child learn how to moderate sweet treats is to encourage their partnership with a healthier food item, such as milk, fruit, or a whole grain food. For example, if you're serving cookies, pair them with milk or berries. Or allow candy with cheese and whole grain crackers. Take advantage of this boundary by teaching it to your child. Over time, he's more likely to adopt this healthy eating habit.

Sample Language: "Sweets are yummy on your tongue, but your body also needs some fuel (nutritious food) to keep it going. I'd like you to have some milk or a cheese stick with those cookies."

No Food in Front of the TV
_____

Eating in front of the TV is associated with mindless eating and weight gain in children, according to a 2015 study in *Obesity* which looked at over 11,000 kindergartners (Peck, 2015). Researchers associated even an hour of television with a 50-60% increased chance of becoming overweight. Why? Sitting around watching TV is a passive, sedentary activity, and likely replaces opportunities for physical activity. Playing on the computer or watching videos on the smart phone may have the same effect.

Setting limits around snacking while passively viewing videos, playing online games, or watching TV may help your child tune in to what she's eating and how much. And this can help her better regulate her appetite and prevent overeating.

Sample Language: "Our rule is no eating in front of screens. Let's pause the TV/game/video while you have your snack and you can restart it afterward."

No Distractions While Snacking

Along the same lines, toys at the table are something parents of younger children may use to help their kids eat, especially those who are picky eaters or who have trouble sitting for a snack. But toys are like iPads or television. They're just another distraction that encourages disengagement with the experience of eating. Ideally, the focus of snack time should be on the experience of eating the snack (which typically takes 10-15 minutes). Distractions extend the snacking timeframe and may interfere with recognizing fullness or satisfaction.

Sample Language: "We have just a few minutes for snack time. Let's focus on enjoying your snack, then we can resume playing (with the toy) when you're done."

SNACKING OUTSIDE OF THE HOME

Mastering boundaries within your home makes it easier to reinforce expectations for snacking outside of your home. Of course, the reality is you have little control over what your child is exposed to or what he eats when you're not around. That being said, you can still give your child the tools to navigate the outside world of snacking.

Desserts, candy, and sugary drinks will not disappear. Nor will school parties, birthday parties, end-of-year celebrations, holiday festivities, and sporting event gatherings. These are prominent in your child's world and will continue to be. While you may have the urge to control them (or may try to), doing so may cause more problems. And that's not good.

For some families, food and unhealthy snacks are a daily obstacle and a major frustration. The sheer number of food decisions can overwhelm and exhaust, especially if you're a family who is trying to balance healthy eating as a priority.

Yet, for your child, it's exciting to see snacks he rarely sees at home. There may be a natural desire to try everything available. Over the years, some of my clients have shared their excitement:

"Kate's mom always has goodies. I can't decide what to eat... I want them all!"

"There are so many desserts and they all look so good..."

"All my favorite foods are at Sam's house. It's hard to choose only one."

While you may dread it when your child gets invited to a friend's house, or a party, or feel extra frustrated when you hear your child has had another cupcake celebration at school, there are some strategies you can teach your child to encourage mindful eating, even when you're not around. For example, remind him of the 90–10 Rule. Encourage your child to save up his *Fun Foods* if he knows there will be an event during the day. If there are several indulgent food items to choose from, encourage your child to look at everything before choosing, then choose the item he cannot leave without eating. Also, suggest your child choose water instead of soda or juice when outside your home.

If your child consistently overdoes it with snacking when

you're not around, it may be time to sit down and have a talk about your expectations, and why they're important to you. Sharing why nutritious snacks help his well-being, and why you want him to choose them can go a long way. Understand your child won't be a perfect eater outside your home (Who is?!). Exploring new foods and flexing the independence muscle are expected and should be celebrated. Don't go overboard with snacking rules outside your home, as this can appear too controlling and drive your child toward unhealthy snacking and sneaking.

Sneak Snacking

I often receive emails about children and teens who sneak snacks. Stories of empty food wrappers discovered in closets or under beds leave parents feeling concerned and looking for help. They wonder if they somehow caused this bad eating habit. It doesn't really matter what the food is, or how old or young the child is, sneaking snacks is disturbing and concerning.

While there is a psychological backbone to sneak snacking, which I'll get into soon, there is also the possibility of physical hunger. Kids who don't get enough to eat or who get empty calories at snack time may still be hungry, driving them to seek more snacks. Your child's brain chemistry may also play a role. The pleasure response in the brain is lit up by highly palatable foods, such as those containing sugar, fat, and salt. These food nutrients trigger feel-good brain chemicals, including dopamine. Once children experience pleasure from eating certain foods, they may feel an urge to eat them again. For instance, the more sweets a child eats, the more potential there will be for increased pleasure and liking, and perhaps cravings for those foods.

Although weight may not be a problem with your child, we have some research to inform us about sneak snacking in children who carry extra weight. A 2016 study in *Appetite* found that parents who monitored their child's intake closely had kids who ate more sweets (Liang, 2016). Likewise, mothers who used psychological control like food restriction had kids who ate more snack foods.

What this means is that if your child experiences too many restrictions on snacks, especially sweet treats, it may create a psychological response of wanting those foods even more. If you're focused on limiting types of foods or the amounts your child is allowed to eat, you might find your child is extra focused on snacking. This psychological response may lead to sneaking.

NIBBLE ON THIS

No doubt, parenting around snacks is a delicate dance. I'll dig more deeply into this aspect in Chapter Nine, but for now, know that boundaries and limits around snacking support your structure and approach to healthy snacking habits. But boundaries can be too restrictive if you're not careful. Find ways to say 'Yes' to your child. For example, *"We're not having any more sweets today, but we can have more tomorrow."* Or, *"We've had our fill of crackers today, but if you're still hungry, I've got bananas or apples."*

When you keep snacks contained, you are setting up the blueprint for healthy snacking habits. You're giving your child the framework to navigate snacking within your home, and without you around. And that will pay off.

Upward and onward! Next, we head into Chapter Six and the letter "S," for *Simple and Easy*. No need to make the job of feeding snacks complicated! I'll help you with lots of ideas around nutritious but simple and easy suggestions for snacks that will satisfy your child (and you!).

Take the challenge!

Try to implement one boundary this week. Stick to it and note your child's responses. Remember, it can take up to two weeks for kids to learn that the new system is here to stay.

SNACKSMART: S

S IS FOR SIMPLE & EASY

Years ago, Debbie discovered Pinterest. She loved getting food ideas and recipes for mealtime. It inspired her to make decadent desserts and healthier snacks. Even though her attempts at making recipes resemble the pictures on Pinterest didn't always work out, she kept at it.

Until one day she hit a wall. "Jill, how do all these other moms do it?" she asked.

"What do you mean?" I asked.

"How do they make food look so good? They're so creative! They must have all the time in the world to bake and cook. I *want* to make things fun and interesting for my kids. I *want* snacks to be exciting and healthy. But I don't have the time or the energy — or even the interest — to do this."

Truth be told, Debbie was torn between wanting to give her children fun, nutritious snacks and the realities of time, effort, and desire, which were in short supply. As a result, she was feeling tension and guilt. Not to mention, she suffered from "comparitis" which left her feeling inadequate.

I had to admit; I felt the same way. "I don't think moms do

this 100% of the time. I think they pick what works for them," I said. "You have my permission to do what works for *you*. Make those fun Pinterest-worthy snacks when you *can*, and when it will reward you and your kids."

Pinterest, Facebook, magazines, and other media can inspire. But they've never been the authority or guide on how to make snacks or any other meal.

In my years of working with families, I've seen more guilt around what we perceive as the standard for meals and snacks for kids: perfectly coifed lunch boxes and from-scratch, healthy snacks. These standards are set, not by health authorities, but by social media outlets and others who may not be in the day-to-day trenches of feeding kids.

From cute cutout snack sandwiches and gourmet food combinations to homemade "healthy" versions of cookies and other treats, they bombard moms everywhere with what they should make in the kitchen. And the underlying message? You should spend your time cooking, baking, shaping, and assembling creative, delicious, inventive, nutritious snacks and meals for your kids. Making food for your kids should be your #1 priority.

Let's be real. These perfect iterations of healthy snacks, while appealing and attractive, aren't always possible or realistic. I think we moms inherently know this, but the pressure to measure up still exists. And where does that lead?

Handing over the granola bar. Letting your kid wander into the pantry and pick chips or crackers for a snack. Making a baggie of Goldfish and letting your child roam around, snack in tow. Stopping at the convenient mart on the way to sports practice.

The guilt you feel may lead to throwing in the towel on snacks. Giving up.

Before we dive deeper in to this chapter, let me be clear: You don't have to make a perfect snack. It doesn't have to be home-made or the perfect combination of healthy foods. Nor does it have to be a clever ensemble or a colorful piece of art. *You do you.* You do what works. I give you permission to let go of the high standards of what a healthy snack *should* look like, and the resulting self-comparisons and constant feelings of not measuring up.

Simple and easy is A-OK. In fact, most kids enjoy snacks when they are straightforward, tasty, and easy to eat. And you'll likely have more success serving easy-to-identify whole foods, anyway.

That's what this chapter is all about: S *is for Simple and Easy.* Here, I'm going to build your toolbox of ideas and inspiration. You won't get Pin-worthy recipes from me (well, maybe a couple). From creative ways to serve snacks to enticing snack combinations, packaged snack ideas and more, this chapter gives you several options so you can focus on what feels right, based on what you have time for and your desires.

For example, you may have more time on the weekends and can make homemade trail mix or bean brownies. Or, during the week, you may have a day when you're running around and need easy, to-go snacks. Given your day, you should be able to navigate your options and select one that works. Of course, I'll showcase real food so that snacks add to the overall nutrition your child gets. And there will be room for treats! But if you need to grab a packaged snack on your way out the door, that's okay too.

Ready to do this?

I Want a Snack Now!

Today's parents face more demands on them than ever before. Twenty-three and a half million moms with children under 18 worked in 2020, according to the U.S. Census Bureau (Christnacht, 2020). They juggled a full- or part-time schedule of work and balanced it with the responsibilities of keeping a home and feeding their family. Many women had a partner to help with these tasks, but a quarter of moms are parenting alone, according to a 2019 Pew Survey (Geiger, 2019).

Over 11 million parents, or about 18%, stayed at home to care for their children in 2016, according to another U.S. Census report (Livingston, 2018). And more dads (6%) are staying at home as the primary caretaker. This doesn't mean the demands on parents are less or fewer. Stay-at-home parents spend more time on childcare and doing housework. And they may also volunteer, chauffeur, and take part in their child's extracurricular experiences.

Some parents face financial constraints that make the food budget a daily concern. Affordability dictates the pantry and refrigerator contents for these families. And let's not forget that they also make snacking decisions based on the child in front of them. If you're dealing with a finicky eater or a kid with strong food preferences, you may be constantly striving to please her.

All this to say the pressures of time, financial resources, and child food preferences influence your daily food decisions at snack time. I think that's a good reason to keep snacks simple and easy so you can get them served quickly.

Here we'll cover some creative strategies to get snacks on the table, keep them nutritious, and 'knock the socks off' your child's excitement about eating them.

. . .

Strategy #1: Creative Cuteness That's Easy

Whip out a knife or a cookie cutter and you've got a leg up on making attractive curiosities at snack time. Food faces on plates, cute animal shapes, and even good ol' geometric shapes like circles and triangles are a hit with lots of kids. Especially young ones.

A 2017 study in *Appetite* showed that preschoolers who played with fruits and vegetables during a hands-on sensory activity ate more fruits and vegetables (even ones they weren't familiar with) later (Coulthard, 2017).

If you're game, play with creating simple snacks using basic shapes that naturally occur in food, or that you can create yourself. For example, think of bread or toast as a canvas for a picture. Even the plate you serve snacks on is a blank slate.

Get basic with geometric shapes like the circles found in crackers, bagels, waffles, and English muffins. Rectangles can be found in cheese blocks and graham crackers. See the square in a deli slice of cheese, a slice of bread, and a waffle? A cheese stick and a whole peeled carrot are cylinders. Take these common shapes found naturally in food and create a bigger picture. Better yet, let your child build it.

Engaging your child with fun pictures, towers, and other constructive elements from food encourages play, which may very well be the path to enjoyable eating. Prepare the food and let your child make a face pattern on a plate. Or, together, make a watermelon pizza, a choo-choo train made of grapes and cheese, or a mini-bagel snowman. Your kid may be more likely to eat that healthy snack.

Strategy #2: Go for Straightforward

Now, if you're shaking your head and thinking, *no way—not my style*, or *my kids are too old for this*, then perhaps the straightforward, do-it-yourself approach is up your alley. You can still make interesting and healthy snacks without the hands-on involvement of your child.

Remember, we're making this easy. But tasty and attractive is riding shotgun. Here are a few ideas to get you started:

Basic Fruit Smoothie

Smoothie Bowls

English Muffin Pizza

Walk-with-Me Taco Packets

Baked Tater Skins

Quick Quesadillas

You can find these recipes (and more!) in the Appendix.

Strategy #3: Pair Packaged Snacks with a Whole Food

Most kids I know enjoy a bag of cheesy crackers or a granola bar. They like the convenience and the "cool" factor of a packaged snack. Their parents like them for the convenience, ease, and ability to placate a whining child. But remember, as we discussed in Chapter Four, packaged snacks or ultra-processed foods may not cover your child's appetite for long and may be short on nutrition.

So how can you make a packaged snack work for your child? Instead of forbidding or avoiding them altogether, make them work by pairing them with a whole food, preferably one with protein, fiber, or healthy fats.

Here are some ideas:

Cheezits + apple slices

Tortilla chips + guacamole

Pretzels + hummus cup

Packaged nuts + milk

Granola bar + cheese stick

Potato chips + applesauce cup

Packaged chocolate chip (or any other kind) cookie + milk

I've got a list of my favorite 'better-for-your-kid' packaged snacks in the Appendix.

Strategy #4: Use the MYO (Make Your Own) Approach

As you will learn in Chapter Ten, during childhood, kids are striving for autonomy with eating and food choices. Not only do they like what they like, they want to have some agency around how it's done. Enter the Make Your Own (MYO) approach.

I'm not suggesting you open the kitchen and say, *Anything goes, have at it!* Not at all. What I'm suggesting is that you set up a snack environment that puts you in charge of the *what* (the food selections) and your child in charge of the *how and which* (the food combinations).

My favorite ways to do this are with a Snack Bar or a Snack Platter.

A Snack Bar is like a dinner bar, smorgasbord, or party scene where the food items being served are lined up. For example, you may serve cereal and milk for snack. Using a Snack Bar approach, you'll set out two different boxes of cereal, a carton of milk, and a small bowl of raspberries and a small bowl of blueberries. Your child takes a small bowl and makes his cereal snack from these items.

A Snack Platter achieves the same result: Your child chooses his snack combination from the items available; however, all the snack options are served on a larger plate. For example, you may place carrot sticks, red pepper slices, a small container of hummus, some cheese cubes, a few pistachios, and a small pile of pretzels on a platter.

You can do both approaches with a single child, but it's even more efficient for parents with multiple children, whether they be siblings or guests.

Snack Bar Ideas

Here are some fun themes and ideas for a MYO Snack Bar:

Build a Cereal Bowl: Use a selection of low sugar cereals, fruit, nuts, seeds, and milk

Top a Tater: Use baked potatoes (they're fast to make in the microwave) and a variety of toppings such as shredded cheese, steamed vegetables, leftover chili, sour cream, and salsa

Perfect Parfaits: Assemble a selection of plain or flavored yogurt, berries or other chopped fruit, jam, granola, dry cereal, nuts, or seeds

Waffles or Toasts with Toppings: Lay out your Snack Bar with toasted whole grain bread or waffles, nut butter, chocolate hazelnut spread, banana slices, blueberries, chocolate chips, and/or crushed nuts.

Snack Platter Combos

What's great about a snack platter is that you can make it themed and well-planned, or just use whatever you have on hand. That it's presented on one platter and there's a variety from which to choose is what's exciting for kids. Here are some themed ideas to get you going:

Italian Snack Platter: Place cut up mozzarella cheese sticks, rolled up salami or other deli meat, sliced red peppers, olives, and bread sticks or crackers on a platter.

Tex-Mex Snack Platter: Combine tortilla chips, yellow pepper slices, guacamole, salsa, shredded cheese, black olives, and bean dip on a platter.

Veggies & More Platter: Serve up carrot sticks, sugar snap

peas, cucumber spears, hummus, and Ranch dressing. If this includes too many veggies, throw some grapes on the platter too.

Fruit & Nuts Platter: Offer apple slices, clementine slices, grapes, whole grain crackers, nut butter, peanuts, cashews, and yogurt-covered pretzels. Add some veggies if you like!

Strategy #5 Healthier Homemade Snacks

Many parents are looking for healthier ways to make sweets and treats. If you enjoy baking, this may be an approach to healthy snacking that speaks to you. One benefit is that you will have more control over the ingredients when you make it yourself. For example, it's easy to cut down the sugar in a cookie recipe, or substitute applesauce for oil in quick breads or brownies.

When my kids were younger, I baked brownies and cookies when I had more time, which was on the weekends. I packaged our treats in individual wrappers and froze them for the week. This took treats off the countertop, kept the portions in check, and ensured they were fresh for an after-school snack, lunch, or dessert.

Some chefs and experts make their living off of upgrading and "healthifying" recipes. That's not me. You'll be able to find a host of ideas and recipes on the internet, but I've culled some of my favorites from my own recipe box and those of my nutrition colleagues. Be sure to look in Appendix at the back of the book for healthy snack recipes, including some of my standbys like Easy Stove-Top Granola, GORP, and fruit leather.

NIBBLE ON THIS

. . .

Simple, easy snacks are possible. Having myriad ways to serve them and make them healthier will keep you in the game and prevent you from giving up. But here's the thing: *You do you.* If you're exhausted and frazzled from working or the demands of parenting, choose the easiest path, like a packaged snack with additional wholesome food. And don't feel guilty about it.

If you have more interest and energy, then explore snack platters or healthier homemade treats. Have fun, explore your creativity, and use snack time as an opportunity to create an adventure with food for your child.

By now, you've learned about the nutrition aspect of healthy snacks, from nutrients and portions to timing and kitchen boundaries. In the next chapters, we're delving into regulating snacks and other, equally important aspects of healthy snacking. In Chapter Seven, you'll learn how to model good snacking habits and monitor your child's eating. As you continue to move through this book, I hope you'll see that healthy snacking involves more than serving up healthy food options. Let's get into the bigger picture around raising a *Smart Snacker*!

Take the Challenge!

Try out a novel way to serve or make snacks this week. Maybe you'll try the Snack Platter or a new recipe. Note how your child responds. If you get a positive response, you have a new tactic in your toolbox! If your child responds negatively, don't lose heart. Try something else. Keep tweaking, you'll get there!

A Bonus Challenge: Snap a shot of your snack and tag me (@the.nourished.child) on Instagram!

7

SNACKSMART: M

M IS FOR MODEL & MONITOR EATING

A nne considered herself a healthy eater. She loved many foods and loved to cook and bring new foods to the family table. She was pretty relaxed about her kids and their eating. She had a good idea of what they ate during the day, even when unexpected food came into their lives. She understood she couldn't make her kids eat, but felt the responsibility to introduce them to a variety of foods. She never got mad when her kids wouldn't try something, told her they traded food, or had an extra treat from a friend. Anne would just take this information into account and adjust her food offerings at home.

Helen was not so relaxed. Nor was she organized about feeding her kids. They were allowed to come in and out of the kitchen and help themselves to snacks. They were also "picky" and demanding about snacks. (She, too, was on the picky side.) And one of her kids was a sneaker, and not completely honest when asked about eating at friends' houses and other venues. All of this made Helen feel like she didn't have a good understanding of the eating habits of her kids, which made her frustrated and more inclined to police their eating. The difference between Anne and Helen was this: One had a good grasp of role modeling and monitoring her kids' eating (Anne) and the other did not (Helen).

In this chapter, I'll explore the letter "M" in the acronym SNACK SMART. M is for *Model and Monitor Eating*. Not only do parents need to be a role model for healthy eating, they need to monitor what their kids eat. Monitoring is important, not only to keep track of overall nutrition, but as a strategy for building healthy snacking habits that last. If you're a "Helen," you'll learn how to be better at monitoring your child's eating; you'll learn to be more of an "Anne," so you can become an excellent guide for your children around eating and snacking.

LIKE PARENT, LIKE CHILD

You probably already know how important it is to be an exemplary role model. From establishing physical activity and sleep habits to using manners in social situations, children look to the adults in their lives to show them the way. Role modeling, especially for food and eating, includes eating healthy foods in front of children and showing enthusiasm for them (even when foods are less preferred).

During the early years, children are learning what, when, and how much to eat based on what they learn from their parents, including attitudes about food, eating, and their food habits, according to a 2007 study by researchers focused on feeding children (Savage, 2007). Parents play a vital role in the experiences children have with food and eating, and several studies link this to eating behaviors and even a child's weight status.

Showing your child how to eat, implanting the norms of your family's diet, and how to interact at the meal table is powerful. We associate role modeling as a positive thing, but it can have a negative side too. For example, if you are "picky," or have a narrow diet, many foods will not appear on the table on enough occasions to allow your child adequate exposure or for positive role modeling, as highlighted in a 2018 study (Scaglioni, 2018).

If you have strong preferences for sweets or highly processed snacks, it's likely you will influence your child to eat them. Or, if you don't eat enough during the day, then binge on snacks mindlessly to compensate, your child will learn those eating patterns. It's almost as if osmosis is occurring; a child naturally absorbs your food selections, eating patterns, and preferences.

Unfortunately, some parents aren't aware of their role modeling tendencies. This is called *unintentional, unhealthy role modeling*, and its influence on children's eating is not fully understood. But as you can imagine, it may have a negative effect on children.

Let's be clear on this. Even though it seems like your child isn't watching you eat, she is. In fact, she's watching more than your eating habits. From how you put on makeup and the clothes you wear, to what you say about your body and whether you are active, your child is taking mental notes on it all. And it's a powerful thing.

Being a role model for how you want your child to eat, exercise, and live shapes his future habits. Most importantly, walk the talk. Be that person who acts like the person you want your child to become: a healthy eater, a *Smart Snacker*, an active person, a good sleeper, a non-dieter, or whatever you deem important to raising the best human you can. In other words, behave the way you want your child to behave.

Role modeling is rooted in day-to-day monotony, so be patient. Its effects accumulate. While you may not notice a positive impact now, have faith you will see it one day, especially if you are consistently trying to be a model of health and wellness.

———

66 Be the model of health you want your child to become.

———

Monitoring: Keeping Track of Your Child's Eating

Monitoring is the frequency with which parents "keep track" of their child's consumption of different foods (particularly sweets, snacks, and high-fat foods), as pointed out by a 2016 review study focused on what it takes to be an effective food parent (Vaughn, 2016). Keeping track of your child's eating has a few benefits, including accounting for nutrients consumed, understanding if they are missing food groups, keeping tabs on sweets and treats, and altering your menu based on your child's eating.

Monitoring what your child eats, how much, and how frequently isn't clear cut. In fact, the research on this topic isn't conclusive. Meaning, monitoring has been shown to promote a healthy diet to a certain point, but too much monitoring may be counterproductive, affecting eating behavior negatively. Ultimately, the optimum level of monitoring may depend on your child's temperament (which we will explore in Chapter Ten), his eating style, and age.

Our friend Anne was good at monitoring her children's eating and made adjustments as the day rolled out. You can probably imagine the opposite scenario: A world where there is no monitoring. Where kids are free to eat what they please and when. Yes, it's an unhealthy scenario for them.

Children need their parents to check in and keep track of eating from time to time, within reason. Think of it this way: if you drive cross-country in a car using a map, periodically you will check the map to make sure you're on the right track. If you don't, you may get lost along the way. Monitoring your child's eating is your way of "checking the map." It allows you to see if your child is headed in the right direction with his food choices and snacking habits.

THE FOOD MONITOR VS. THE FOOD COP

As you probably surmised, Helen didn't monitor her kids very well. As a result, she sometimes felt things were out of her control. To take back the reins, she did what many parents do: She controlled every bite of food, especially sweets and treats. What was worse, she vacillated between letting her kids have full access to the kitchen (and treats) and placing tight controls on foods in her home. This made the situation worse because it confused her kids. They sensed an unpredictability around food access and sneaked snacks.

Helen morphed into a food cop, patrolling every morsel of food eaten. It was the only way she could contain and control her kids' eating. In a nutshell, she didn't trust her kids with food. Over the years, I've encountered parents like Helen who believed they needed to control or restrict the food their kid eats. If they didn't, the child would eat too much, or the wrong foods and gain weight. Foods like candy or chips became "forbidden" and scarce. This is known as *food restriction* or *restrictive feeding practices.* Although parents believe they're helping their child, being too restrictive with food may cause more problems later in life.

The research in this area, particularly around snacking, points out that being restrictive, or too controlling with food, is consistently associated with *more* snacking among children (Blaine, 2017). This is especially true when there are unhealthy foods like sweets and treats present in the home.

What Is Food Restriction?

Food restriction is limiting food consumption intending to control the eating habits, weight, or caloric intake of a child. It shows up in different ways, including eliminating or strictly limiting access to certain foods, like desserts; or limiting the amount of food eaten; or using modified foods (i.e., fat-free or sugar-free) to control calorie intake.

BLURRED LINES BETWEEN MONITORING AND RESTRICTION

Tightly controlling food or policing it is not monitoring. Monitoring is an awareness of what your child is eating as he moves through his day. Restriction is taking action to control how much or what your child is eating. That's a big difference.

As you've learned in the Liang study in the Sneak Snacking section, restriction may have negative effects on a child's eating, food choices, and weight. Mothers who used psychological control such as pressure to eat certain foods and restriction of other foods had kids who ate *more* snack foods. These parents blurred the line between monitoring and restriction, leaning towards patrolling food consumption. When sweets are taboo, your child may want to eat them more. It's reverse psychology.

A child's perception of what's going on in her food world matters. If a child perceives some foods are being restricted, then it's likely they will respond accordingly with increased attention to those foods.

"... children who perceive their mothers as using more coercive practices to reduce their overeating, or who perceive more psychological control from their mothers eat more beyond satiety," stated June Liang, the study author. Translated: If your child thinks you're too controlling or restrictive with food, it may encourage your child to eat more.

Another point rings true from the scientific evidence on restriction: Using restrictive feeding practices regularly can foster a loss of appetite awareness. Children may lose their sense of hunger and fullness. This may lead to overeating, especially when there are sweets and treats in the home, and especially when kids aren't under the watchful eye of their parent.

———

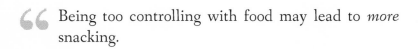 Being too controlling with food may lead to *more* snacking.

———

Taking a Guilt-Free Stance on Snacking

If you're inclined to scroll through your social media platforms, pick up the latest magazine, or chat with your friends about how your kid eats, you may feel pangs of guilt. Comparing your kid to the high standards of wholesome, organic, farm-fresh, natural, preservative-free, and non-GMO eating that the world would have you believe is happening in every other home will make you feel less, if not guilty, for sure.

Guilt is a self-conscious emotion, causing many who feel it to reflect. It's an uncomfortable emotion, but it can spur change. Experts believe this is the positive aspect of guilt. For parents and feeding kids, guilt centers on a failure to feed their child the way they think they're supposed to. "Mom guilt" is complicated, because parents don't *intentionally* feed their kids poorly.

Experts suggest that those who feel guilt try to soothe this feeling in one of two ways: They try to make it up to the person who was wronged, or do something for others to ease their guilty feelings. Yet, other research has shown that guilt may positively influence decision-making. It can lead you to be more generous, for example.

How does this play out in feeding kids? When parents feel guilty about what their kids snack on, for example, it may motivate negative feeding, such as food restriction, or pressure to eat. Parents may use this to correct their kids' poor eating habits. On the other hand, guilt may spur generosity. For example, *I'm the reason you have bad eating habits, so I'm going to allow other privileges to make up for it.*

Kids may also feel guilty. Experts say that kids as young as two years old experience guilt and try to make up for it. Some kids may feel guilty about what they like to eat. For example, many kids enjoy sweets and treats, some feel soothed by certain foods, and others turn to food to comfort difficult emotions. When children hear comments about how bad the foods they enjoy eating are, or how unhealthy it is to eat them, they may feel guilty. This may mess up their self-image, their relationship with food, and the ability to self-regulate their eating.

I think what's helpful is to be compassionate with yourself. If you're feeling guilty about your child's eating habits, think about whether things were out of your control. For example, did the outside world expose your child to sweets and treats, or was life crazy when your kids were younger and you were just getting by?

Do you know more now than you did then? As we grow in our parenting, we get better because our knowledge is deeper. Are your standards of yourself influenced by outside forces, and/or are they unattainable for you or your kids? If you're looking to others to define a standard of snacking or eating for your family, maybe you should stop listening to them. It's *your* family, not theirs.

And take care not to make your kid feel guilty about the foods he enjoys eating. Eating enjoyment is a behavior you're trying to cultivate, not squash.

One thing I know is that kids change and develop. Their taste buds grow up and become more open to new cuisines and flavors. What they like to eat as kids may still be liked as an adult, but they learn to eat for broader reasons than just flavor. I know this for myself, and my own kids, and the families with which I've worked. Hang in there! If guilt is grabbing you daily, take a step back and reflect on why. What can you change? What can you give up? Guilt should be top of your list.

OTHER FEEDING PRACTICES THAT CAN CHANGE YOUR CHILD'S SNACKING

While food restriction and increased snacking are connected, there are some other feeding practices I want to mention before we move on. Remember, feeding is the interaction around food, not the food itself. Some practices I want to highlight are catering, rewarding, and pressure to eat, as these may change your child's snack preferences and appetite regulation.

Catering: Also known as short-order cooking, catering is characterized by making a child what he wants to eat. Often, short-order cooks make separate meals to please certain family members, usually a picky eater. One survey found that 80% of parents with picky eaters felt they had little control over their child's food choices and their eating. Seventy-five percent of parents gave in to their picky eater's requests for food.

When parents become short-order cooks, it tells a child he can have whatever he wants to eat. Sometimes, poor behavior like whining or tantrums are tied up in catering, making parents take the easier road: making something that will please their child.

The evidence on catering tells us it limits a child's willingness to try new foods, and may limit the nutritional quality of the diet. A 2009 study in the *International Journal of Behavioral Nutrition and Physical Activity* found that short-order cooking discouraged consumption of nutritious foods like fruit, veggies, and dairy products. From a snacking standpoint, catering may influence what your child will snack on. For example, if you want to offer a vegetable-based snack option, but your child *won't* eat veggies, you will face resistance. If you find you're in the throes of short-order cooking for a picky eater, my book *Try New Food: How to Help Picky Eaters Taste, Eat & Like New Foods* takes a thorough analysis into the actions you can take to remedy your situation.

Rewarding: Rewarding with food is also called *Instrumental Feeding* in the scientific literature on feeding kids. It's a strategy used by parents to manipulate or control their child's eating behavior or food intake by using incentives, which may be food-based (candy or dessert) or non-food-based (stickers or praise). Often, sweets are used to reward children for good behavior, trying a new food, or eating a certain amount of food. Sweet food rewards may reinforce an existing preference for sweets, build an inclination toward sugary foods, and may reduce your child's willingness to accept healthier snacks (Johnson, 2016).

Why do parents use food rewards? Because bribing kids to eat is effective. In the short-term, anyway. Tell Bobby he can have a brownie after dinner if he eats all of his broccoli, or takes five bites of chicken, or cleans his plate, and more often than not, you'll get a willing eater (even if he's not hungry or doesn't like that food). When you use a food reward, especially sweets, you may see an immediate result: a child who eats more, tries new food, or eats healthy food.

The research tells us there's more to the story, however. In a 2016 study out of Aston University in the UK, researchers looked at children aged 3 to 5 years and the feeding practices their parents used. They followed up with these children when they were 5 to 7 years old. What they found? Children were more likely to be emotional eaters at that age if their parents had reported using food as a reward when they were younger (Ellis, 2016).

Another 2017 review study in *Appetite* recommended, based on the evidence we have to date, that "... food-based rewards should not be used in order to make children eat every day, well-accepted foods" (DeCosta, 2017).

The bottom line? Using food rewards like sweets may decrease the preference for the foods kids already like, while increasing their preference for the reward food (often a sweet food).

You may wonder about other rewards that aren't food. There is some evidence for using non-food rewards for kids (i.e., stickers) to help children get over the fear of, or resistance to, trying a new food. Since tasting a new food is required in helping kids learn to like new foods, non-food rewards can incentivize children to taste them. However, using non-food rewards may undermine a child's ability to develop a natural drive and motivation to try new food. Use caution with them. If you sense it isn't working well, then adjust your course of action.

Pressure to eat: Some parents pressure their children to take another bite of food or eat more, hoping to motivate their child to eat a certain food, a certain amount, or try something new. Pressure to eat is one of the most common tactics parents use to influence their children's eating. Yet, most parents will confess that it doesn't really work. Luckily, I have some data to help you understand what's really going on.

First, researchers have found that kids who are reminded to eat (called prompting or nagging) and pushed to eat more (known as pressuring or forcing) may eat more, and perhaps too much. It's suggested by several studies that pressure to eat causes disruption in a child's ability to self-regulate his eating. The inherent sense of fullness following a meal or snack is dulled, which disturbs the instinct to stop eating.

Furthermore, experts postulate that poor self-regulation and *Eating in the Absence of Hunger* (defined as eating for non-hunger reasons like emotions or boredom) is connected to the development of unhealthy weight and childhood obesity.

However, a 2018 longitudinal study in *Appetite* emphasizes that it's not just pressure to eat that may cause a disturbance in self-regulation, but the intent, tone, and manner by which pressure is used, that may be more important (Galindo, 2018).

Second, with pressure to eat, some kids experience it differently, especially those who are picky eaters. A study in *Appetite* found that children experienced "early satiety" (also known as early fullness) and didn't eat more when forced or pressured to do so. They stopped eating early in the meal and ate less overall because of feeling full. This, they felt, may relate to a physiological or psychological response triggering an early release of satiety hormones. Some of their study subjects became pickier. The researchers also showed kids may develop a dislike for the foods they feel pressured to eat, like vegetables (Galloway, 2006).

What about the type of pressure parents use, and how that influences kids' eating? For example, the above 2018 study in *Appetite* reinforced that pressure to eat new foods was tied to eating when not hungry. Interestingly, though, pressure to eat familiar foods didn't have this affect.

Other research looks at the chicken and egg argument: Are parents pushing their kids to eat because they're fussy eaters? A 2017 study in *Physiology & Behavior* examined moms and young children, finding that picky eating predicted the use of pressure to eat. Translated: Parents use pressure to eat as a response to picky eating (Jansen, 2017).

Another 2014 study in *Appetite* looked at 8- and 9-year-old kids and their level of anxiety and whether they perceived pressure at the table. They found kids with symptoms of anxiety and depression more readily perceived pressure to eat from their parents (Houldcroft, 2014).

Last, that earlier study of college students revealed that pressure in childhood led to problematic eating in young adulthood (Ellis, 2016).

As a parent, it's hard to know if you're complicating things by pressuring your child to eat, because each child is different. Encouragement may not bother some kids and, hence, they eat more food. Obviously, this may lead to overeating and a poor ability to regulate their appetite. Other kids may dig in their heels, offended by pressure, and becoming more picky or contrary about eating. Both outcomes lead to disruptions in appetite regulation.

You can see how these feeding tactics and interactions are a powerful influence on shaping your child's snacking habits. While monitoring is favorable and restriction is detrimental, it's still important to be aware of *all* the interactions around feeding your child, regardless of whether it's meals or snacks.

THE ROLE OF COMMUNICATION AND MONITORING

When I explain monitoring to parents, I emphasize the mental aspect of it. It's the inside job of checks and balances parents use to make future decisions about food offerings. For example, if your child comes home from a friend's house and tells you about all the candy he ate, you'll probably adjust any plans you had for dessert that evening. This is monitoring at its best: Using the information you have to make better food decisions later.

One of the most powerful ways to use monitoring is to explain to your child why you've decided what you have. Such as, "Tommy, it sounds like you had more candy at Jack's house today, so I'm going to reschedule our dessert tonight for tomorrow night." Communicating your "why" can teach and reinforce a healthy balance of foods.

As parents, we have to say no, but how we say it can be the fundamental change in getting your child to comply with your stance on the matter. I encourage you to communicate your "no" in a way that has promise. "Not right now" means "yes, in the future." This tells your child that later he can have that candy or dessert, and this may qualm his unrest.

"No" without a reason, or with no anticipation of future

access, can frustrate a child. Here are a few ways to say "No" nicely:

When your child asks for snacks (and he's not hungry, or just ate)

"The kitchen is closed right now, so I can't get you another snack. But, the good news is that it will be open at 3:00 p.m.—in just a bit."

When your child asks for unplanned sweets

"These are special occasion foods and guess what? Today isn't a special occasion day... but this weekend is! We can have dessert then. I, for one, can't wait!"

"That's not on the menu for today. Let's look for a time when we can include them."

When your child doesn't like what you're offering for snack time

"You're not fond of this snack? I tell you what, why don't you write down a list of your favorite snacks and I will try to work those in over the next week or two."

When your child complains about food

"Boy, the complaining about your snack is really hard for me to hear. I work really hard to make nutritious food available for this family. Let's stop complaining and be more proactive. Would you write some snacks you want me to purchase at the grocery store, please? That would really help me know what to buy next time."

. . .

When your child is melting down because you said "no" to a food request

"Oh, honey, I can see that you aren't happy." (Smile, give a brief hug, and move on.)

When your child refuses to eat

"This is the snack offering for today. I'm sorry you don't like it, but I'm sure you can find something here to eat."

Note, these responses work well for general eating, as well!

MONITORING IN AND OUT OF THE HOME

It's accepted among health experts that children do a good job of eating what they need to grow well and develop when they receive a balance of foods to support healthy growth and development. Without a knowledge of food balance, it will be harder to monitor your child's eating. (If this is something you struggle with, my program *The Nourished Child Blueprint* can help you master this area of nutrition.)

In the home, you have more control and it's easier to monitor your child's eating. A food system that emphasizes a healthy balance of nutritious food, coupled with an eating schedule that supplies this food regularly, makes it apparent when things tip in the wrong direction.

Outside of your home, though, is a different story. Children are exposed to many foods and they must learn to navigate them without their parents. Some of these environments, such as school, sports, after-school activities, and other gatherings can be a challenge to monitor.

Here are a few tips for monitoring your child's eating when they aren't with you:

Communicate Casually about Food

Encourage open communication about your child's day, including what he ate. I think it's best to be curious and not too focused on a specific food, or how much was eaten, but give attention to the experience. How did the food taste? Who did you eat with? Why did you like this food? Have you had that before?

Lead with curiosity and don't be too intense, worried, or negative about your child's choices or behaviors. Remember, you can alter the food plan at home.

Teach and Use the 90–10 Rule

Remember the 90–10 Rule (Chapter Two) is a way to allow sweets and treats in the diet without letting them take over and crowd out healthy foods. At a minimum, this "rule" separates indulgent foods from nutritious foods, which encourages your child to sift and sort food on his own. Over time, the idea is to let your child self-correct and manage his own food balance, especially with sweets and treats.

Include Your Child in the Solution to Challenges

Kids do well when they are part of the solution. While the 90–10 Rule can be part of the solution, it's good to work with your child to solve eating problems, like sneaking snacks or overeating at parties. For example, sit down with your child and ask, *"What should we do about dessert since you had some already today?"*

Or, *"I noticed you took some crackers into your bedroom. We have a rule about no food upstairs. What's going on?"* Partnering with your child shows him you respect and value his input.

Helen had to come to terms with her role in her children's eating. She was too controlling and hadn't mastered the technique of monitoring. You may need to do the same. Check your role in your child's eating behaviors. Are you helping or contributing to the problem?

Remember, it's natural for kids to be excited about food, especially foods that they don't see often, or that might be tightly controlled. If your child goes nuts with sweets at parties, maybe they're too scarce in your home. Or, if sneaking snacks is a problem, maybe your kid is hungrier than you realize and you need to make snacks more satisfying.

Nibble on This

I hope you can see that monitoring your child's eating is an important part of raising a *Smart Snacker*, but it can also be a slippery slope. For some parents, it's easy to slide into controlling behaviors, and as you've learned, this may backfire and create other eating issues.

Monitoring at its best helps you be flexible with snacks and adjust your feeding strategy based on what and how your child is eating.

Next, in Chapter Eight, I'll discuss the letter "A," which stands for *Appetite Awareness*. Here, we'll explore the appetite regulators, the concept of physical hunger versus "head hunger," how to support mindful eating, and why snacks can be your ally.

Take the Challenge!

Take one day and monitor what your child is eating from the start of the day to the end. Did you make an adjustment to your food and feeding plan?

S N A C K S M A R T: A

A IS FOR APPETITE RULES

Welcome to Chapter Eight, where I help you understand appetite regulation and why it's so important to snacking.

As a parent, one of the most important things you can do to influence healthy snacking is to support your child's appetite awareness. Yet there are many obstacles that stand in your way.

Here, we'll build upon the basics I touched on in Chapter One, differentiating between physical hunger and what I call "head" hunger. I'll also discuss how feeding and taste influences appetite, and wrap up with tips for encouraging your child to be more mindful with snacking.

As a mom of four kids, one of my goals has always been to instill a good sense of appetite and an ability to regulate it. I want my kids to stop eating when they're full and know when they need to eat based on their hunger cues. I know how the world makes it harder to instill a good sense of appetite awareness. When food cues and eating opportunities are *everywhere,* it's easier to ignore our internal appetite cues and rely on outside influences that tell us to eat or not. Not only that, constant distractions make eating mindlessly a real danger.

Did you know that when kids stop eating before they've finished everything on their plate, there's a good chance they're listening to their body cues? Yet, some parents aren't happy when a child walks away from an incomplete snack or meal. Alternatively, when a child can't stop eating snacks, it may be a sign that she's not tuned in to her appetite cues.

Why does all this appetite stuff matter? Because how well your child listens to her body and responds to its signals predicts how much and how well she will eat. And that affects her nutritional status and body weight. To highlight this, let's look at two girls, Taylor and Beth.

Taylor was always hungry. Even after a meal, she was ready for a snack right away. Taylor was a "live to eat" kind of girl, looking for her next opportunity to eat, with little credence to whether or not she was hungry. Beth was the opposite. She often stated she was full after eating and didn't seem to ask for food between meals and snacks. She was an "eat to live" kind of girl, eating when she was hungry. The fundamental difference between these two is one child is conscious of her appetite and leads with that, while the other child is not. Can you guess who's who?

Taylor was *out of touch* with her appetite and relied on external cues and her emotions to dictate eating. Beth, on the other hand, was *in tune* with her appetite. She recognized when she was hungry and while eating, could sense satiety (a sense of fullness) creeping in, which cued her to stop.

Appetite 101: Physical Hunger & Satiety

We all experience hunger differently. Sure, there are physical signs of hunger. Tummy growling, light-headedness, headache, or weakness. Even crankiness. That's me. I get cranky. So does my daughter. But have you ever stopped to think about what's behind the physical experience of hunger? Or what happens when you feel full?

The body's ability to regulate appetite is like a theater production. From nutrients acting on the gut to hormones signaling areas of the brain, it turns out the result—feeling hungry or full—involves a cast of characters acting out an elaborate stage show. Although I introduced you to the broad concept of appetite regulation in Chapter One, here, I'm detailing it so you have a keen sense of how it influences your child's eating.

Let's start with the basics. Appetite is controlled by several factors, including hormones and nutrients. These come from the gut and interact with the central nervous system (CNS), specifically the hypothalamus and the brain stem, telling them how much energy we have in our body.

When the brain perceives that we have enough energy in our body, it fires off hormones that suppress eating. When it perceives we haven't eaten enough or have low energy stores, it signals hunger. We call this central regulation. In a very basic sense, hormones signal hunger, which leads to eating. After eating, hormones fire and signal fullness.

Simple, right?

Not exactly. This is where it gets more complicated. Let's dive in deeper.

———

Hunger, Satisfaction, and Fullness

Physical hunger is the body sensation that triggers a desire to eat. Symptoms of physical hunger include stomach growling, headache, fatigue, low energy, and mood swings.

Head hunger is thinking you're hungry, which may also trigger a desire to eat. Boredom, memories of eating, emotional impulses (sadness or celebration, for example), and habits or routines around eating can be reasons for head hunger. Head hunger is also called *Eating in the Absence of Hunger*.

Satisfaction is when you're no longer feeling hungry and not yet feeling full. It's somewhere in between hunger and fullness. This sensation can occur while eating.

Fullness is feeling the stomach is full. It may be an uncomfortable feeling. The signs of fullness include distended belly, feeling sleepy, impaired movement, feeling ill, or generalized discomfort.

———

THE GUT HORMONES

Two hormones, ghrelin and leptin, are the main hormonal appetite regulators. Hunger begins with a dip in blood sugar after a period has passed without eating. This alerts the brain to tell the stomach to secrete the hunger hormone, ghrelin.

Ghrelin increases appetite. It's made in the gut and tells the brain it's time to eat. It's easiest to remember what ghrelin does by thinking about the first three letters of its spelling, "ghr," pronounced *grrrr*, just like the word *growl*.

Fat cells make the other main appetite hormone called leptin. Leptin circulates in the bloodstream and tells the brain you have enough energy and fat to do everyday activities. It tells the brain you're full and decreases appetite signals. However, leptin can be a trickster. When leptin levels decrease, like when you lose weight or don't eat enough, it tells the brain you're *starving*. This message stimulates the body to drive leptin levels back up, which spurs ghrelin and a sense of hunger, leading you to eat more. This meets the body's goal of raising leptin levels back to your personal norm.

Ghrelin and leptin dance together to make sure the body has enough energy. That's their primary objective. They are constantly balancing each other between hunger and fullness. But they are not alone.

Several other hormones tell the body it's full, as well. Let's take a quick review of some of them:

Peptide YY is a hormone produced in direct response to the calorie intake of a meal or snack. A lot of calories consumed will produce a lot of peptide YY, shutting off your appetite. Peptide YY is a satiety signal, telling the body it's full.

Glucagon-Like Peptide-1 (GLP-1) is also a satiety signal. It tells the pancreas to release insulin after eating, inhibiting food intake.

Cholecystokinin (CCK) inhibits food intake by acting on the brain stem. It's released from the gut after eating and stimulates organs to digest food.

Insulin is also a hormone released by the pancreas. It keeps blood sugar levels stabilized, which reduces hunger spikes.

As I said, it's a theater production, and the plot thickens. Let's head to the brain next.

THE REWARD CENTER OF THE BRAIN

Food is rewarding. It's well known that the reward circuit of the brain interacts with several systems, including opioids, the dopaminergic system, endocannabinoids, and serotonin. We also know the pleasure response in the brain is turned on by highly palatable foods, such as those containing sugar, fat, and salt. These nutrients trigger feel-good brain chemicals. Once we experience pleasure from eating certain foods, we remember and may feel an urge to eat them again. Therefore, some people feel "addicted" to foods like sweets and feel they have no control over themselves in their presence.

Seeing palatable food (or food that looks delicious) may also trigger a desire to eat, even when hunger is absent. That's why the smorgasbord spread of desserts are hard to pass up, even when you're full. A fond memory of an eating experience or a food can do the same. Pumpkin pie on Thanksgiving or the neighbor's chocolate chip cookies can stimulate the reward center of the brain and spur appetite. All this is to say, food itself and the experience of eating can spur appetite.

NUTRIENTS AND GROWTH ALSO IMPACT APPETITE

· · ·

As I mentioned, nutrients have an influence on appetite. As you learned in Chapter Two, the nutrients protein, fat, and fiber are filling. These alone may induce a sense of fullness and satiety. Other nutrients, like sugar, aren't so filling and leave kids at risk of feeling hungry before they should be. *Smart Moms* will use filling nutrients when planning snacks to help their kids feel full and satisfied and ward off early hunger.

But, as you may suspect, appetite regulation doesn't end with hormones and food. There are some other factors you need to understand, especially the impact of growth. The dynamic process of physical growth triggers hunger and prompts children to eat. During the two biggest growth spurts in childhood—infancy and adolescence—you'll see an increase in appetite. That's because appetite follows what's going on with growth.

For example, the teenager eats a lot because he is in a growth spurt. If you have a teen, you know this already. But sometimes parents fear this uptick in appetite, afraid it signals bad eating habits or a path to unwanted weight gain. However, when you understand how your child's appetite works with the growth process, you'll see the harmony between the two and worry less.

Children Know How to Regulate Their Appetite

We are all born with a natural sense of hunger, an ability to sense it, and a desire to quench it. Babies expressly tell us when they need to eat. They cry. When they're full, they pull off the breast or turn away from the bottle. Babies push food out of their mouths, throw it on the floor, or bat the spoon away. These are all signs of satisfaction or fullness.

This is self-regulation in its purest form. All the signals are primed and firing on time. The theater production is in full swing and operating beautifully, so to speak. And then real food enters the picture. Babies start solid foods around six months. No doubt, the desire to feed a baby and have it eat well is strong. Parents are invested in this journey, but sometimes they get over-involved, encouraging their little one to take more bites of food, or finish eating everything. These feeding interactions can disarm a child's internal appetite regulation. For instance, when parents encourage more food intake, like eating that last spoonful of baby food, a child's natural sense of fullness can be overridden. Although these little pushes to eat begin in infancy, they don't stop there.

(If you have a baby and are starting solids, my book *The Smart Mom's Guide to Starting Solids* will help you succeed in this stage!)

THE ROLE OF FEEDING IN APPETITE REGULATION

No parent wants to interfere and mess up their child's internal appetite regulation. Not intentionally, anyway. Therefore, it's important for you to understand how powerful your daily feeding interactions can be. *Responsive feeding* is the lingo describing the back-and-forth relationship between a parent and child that exists around feeding and eating. Specifically, responsive feeders understand their child's hunger or fullness cues and respond appropriately to them.

For example, your child wakes up and states he's hungry. You feed him. He eats and stops on his own. You end the meal. This is responsive feeding at its core: your child leads with his appetite and you respond appropriately to it.

Non-responsive feeding is the opposite. It goes something like this: your child comes home from preschool and is grumpy, tired, and seems to be hungry, but you hold him off because it isn't time for lunch yet. When lunch time comes, he eats fast, fills up after a few minutes, and stops. But you want him to finish, so you keep nagging him to take more bites and threaten to take away TV for the afternoon if he doesn't eat more.

Non-responsive feeding plays out at all ages. For example, if there are long periods between meals or not enough calories or nutrients, your child can experience intense hunger during the day. This hunger may cause disturbances in his ability to regulate his eating, potentially causing him to overeat or make poor food choices. Alternatively, when kids are made to eat everything on their plate, this may disarm their "full" signal, leading them to consume too much food.

Researchers believe when we use responsive feeding in infancy and beyond, children are better at self-regulating their food intake and they eat more food variety. We associate these behaviors with a healthy body weight.

On the flip side, researchers also see that when non-responsive feeding is used, children are not as good at regulating their appetite and eating (they don't tune in to their body signals as well and may struggle with overeating or undereating), and this may contribute to weight problems.

Although we like to think children are great at self-regulating their food consumption, many kids just aren't very good at it. The feeding interaction is one area where I believe you can help. Later, I'll give you some tips to help you teach and preserve the hardwired appetite regulation system with which your child was born.

HEAD HUNGER: EATING IN THE ABSENCE OF HUNGER

· · ·

As you may suspect, not all kids eat because they're physically hungry. For instance, your child just ate dinner (a good one), but states he's hungry 30 minutes later. Physically, it's unlikely he's truly hungry, but according to him, he is. His head is telling him to eat. Or, what scientists call *Eating in the Absence of Hunger* (EAH), a term that describes eating (typically highly palatable foods) when not hungry (Lansigan, 2015).

The tendency towards EAH develops between the ages of five and nine when a greater awareness of food and external triggers to eat become more prominent. For example, party treats and social eating may trigger EAH.

Why do kids eat when they're not physically hungry? Well, the reasons vary:

- Your child may be out of touch with body signals related to eating (or has a poor awareness of hunger and fullness cues)
- Your child may eat because food looks good, was previously enjoyed or liked, others are eating it, or it's a scarce or tightly regulated food (also known as a heightened response to food)
- Your child may be impulsive around food (called low inhibitory control)
- Your child may eat to calm or comfort his feelings (eats for emotional reasons)
- Your child may eat because of a perception that there is nothing else to do (also known as boredom)
- Your child eats because food was tightly controlled or off limits and is now available (a reaction to restrictive feeding practices)

Of course, helping your child tune in to their appetite and eat (mostly) for hunger is the goal. Why? Because *Eating in the Absence of Hunger* is associated with extra weight gain in boys and girls under the age of twelve. Your goal is to sustain and maintain that internal regulation system with which your child was born. There will always be external triggers for eating, but these shouldn't be the primary reasons.

Teaching your child about physical hunger is an important step toward helping him develop an internal sense of when to eat and when to stop eating. This is something that can start in the early years, but it's an ongoing endeavor. Early on, you can use terms like 'hungry belly' and 'happy belly' to help your toddler associate the feelings of hunger and fullness cues.

As your child gets older, encourage him to pay attention to his physical cues by asking: *What is your body telling you?* This will not only tie eating to appetite cues, but it will reinforce them and build a memory of these sensations. Another important topic is to identify emotional triggers for eating. When your child is sad, disappointed, lonely, or stressed, it's okay to acknowledge that these emotions are uncomfortable. Encourage your child to talk to someone about those feelings. Communicating emotions is a healthy way to deal with them. Turning to food to soothe or numb strong, negative emotions is not.

How to Support Your Child's Appetite Regulation

As you can imagine, there are several ways to support your child's natural inclination to recognize hunger and fullness. Here are some easy, basic things you can think about and take action with as you feed your child:

. . .

Look for Signs of Real Physical Hunger

Growing children are hungry. But bored children may appear hungry as well. Sort this out and know the difference so you can help your child tune into his body better. Remember, growth is a powerful predictor of hunger. If your child is in a growth spurt, expect hunger to spike and eating to increase.

Stay Ahead of Hunger

Half the battle of managing hunger in children is staying ahead of it. Remember the guidance you received in Chapter One about timing of eating? Strategically plan snacks to occur between meals so that intervals without food don't extend beyond 3–4 hours. Skipping snacks can prompt overeating later on.

Use Filling Nutrients

Remember the power of protein, fiber, and fat: They induce fullness. Use wholesome foods that naturally offer these nutrients such as 100% whole grains, fruits, and vegetables for fiber; dairy products, lean meats, eggs, nuts, and beans for some protein; and healthy fats like avocado, olive oil, nuts, and seeds.

Start On the Right Foot

I know this book is about snacking, but snacks and meals work together. Start the day off with a nutritious breakfast. It starts the body's "engine" and sets the pattern for eating at regular intervals. Studies show that kids who skip breakfast may overeat later in the day. And believe me, that can affect snacking habits.

Putting It Together: Snacking Mindfully

One of the biggest challenges about snacking is that it often happens mindlessly; meaning, kids snack without thinking or registering whether or not they're hungry. As a result, the amounts they eat may be excessive.

You want your child to pay attention to food when he's eating, so he can fully enjoy it and be aware of his body responses to it, specifically, his satisfaction or fullness levels. Awareness builds better self-regulation, and that's the goal.

To build on supporting your child's appetite regulation, here are some super-practical ways to help your child pay attention to what and how much he eats:

Keep Snacks at the Table

We talked about keeping snacks contained in Chapter Five. I want you to maintain a typical spot for snacking. I like to see kids eating in the kitchen, as it minimizes other distractions and allows kids to focus on eating. This builds in more awareness and allows for food conversations more naturally.

Pay Attention to the Food Details

When kids are snacking, don't be afraid to chat about the details of the foods they are eating. What does it taste like? Spicy or sweet? Salty or bland?

What does it feel like? Is it crunchy or mushy? Wet or dry? These food conversations can teach your child a new language to describe food.

Another fun mindfulness experiment is to play with a piece of chocolate. Ask your child to close his eyes and let the chocolate slowly melt in his mouth. What does he notice? How long does it take? Does it feel or taste different?

Play with slowing down the eating process. Paying more attention can encourage more mindfulness.

Talk about Hunger and Satisfaction

In my experience, some kids are clueless about what their bodies are experiencing in relation to eating. They don't know that crankiness may signal hunger. Or that a spike in energy may be a clue they've eaten enough. When kids don't recognize their body sensations, they may use external signals as the regulators of their appetite. They're more inclined to use "head" hunger or external cues as a guide for eating. As you already know, we want kids to pay attention to their physical signs. You can help your child connect the dots, reinforcing the sensations and behaviors associated with hunger and satisfaction. This will reinforce your child's attention to his internal cues rather than external ones.

Let the Chips Fall

When your child skips his snack because he's too busy playing, you need not rescue him an hour later with another snacking opportunity. In fact, it's better you don't. Let your child experience the consequences of not eating (hunger), as it will reinforce the physical sensation of hunger and imprint that feeling for the future.

Likewise, connect the dots when your child overeats. Tie the feeling of discomfort to the behavior of eating too much. Let the chips fall. Allowing the natural consequences of your child's choices will go a long way to reinforce his appetite signals like hunger or fullness and help him regulate his eating better.

. . .

NIBBLE ON THIS

Appetite, and regulating it, is also a struggle for many adults. The plethora of external cues for eating, plus a history of eating habits, makes it harder to be mindful and aware of our own eating. You can prevent this from happening to your child by helping him get a grip on hunger, satisfaction, and fullness.

When your child understands his own appetite, he'll be better able to regulate it himself. Of course, this is a work in progress. As you've learned, there can be many barriers to overcome. One significant obstacle is feeding. I want you to understand and get on top of your feeding interactions so they support your child in his healthy snacking habits.

I'll discuss this in the next chapter, *R is for Responsible Feeding*. In it, I'll teach you how to be more diplomatic in feeding, cover some negative feeding practices parents fall prey to, and give you some fun ways to feed snacks while encouraging self-sufficiency and autonomy.

Take the Challenge!

Do an exercise with your child that promotes appetite awareness and mindfulness: Talk about physical hunger, head hunger, satisfaction, and fullness and take the time to describe the characteristics of food such as flavor, texture, or odor. Try the chocolate exercise!

SNACKSMART: R

R IS FOR RESPONSIVE AND FLEXIBLE

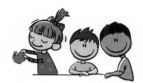

When I was a younger mother and my kids were little, snack time was a production. I treated it like mealtime, even though it was of shorter duration and included smaller servings. In my kitchen, I had a large island countertop. We had wooden stools made for children. They had a semicircular back so that the kids wouldn't topple over backward when they sat in them. My kids sat on these stools for breakfast, lunch, and most dinners, and for snack time, puzzles, and art activities. You could say my kitchen was the 'heart of the home' and where many of our daily activities took place.

I would announce, "It's time for a snack!" and my four kids would come running to the kitchen and climb onto their stools. I'd have a bowl of fruit, which I would hand to one child and instruct her to pass it along to the next. I'd have a plate of cheese and crackers and start that at the opposite end of the counter with a different child. And I'd pass out cups of water. Each child would pick what they wanted for their snack based on what I offered that day.

Sure, sometimes I'd get a *"But I wanted yogurt!"* My

response would be something like *"Oh, I'm sorry. That's not on the menu for today. We can have that tomorrow though!"*

Or, occasionally, I'd hear, *"But I don't like this snack."* I'd say as I smiled at my child, *"Ah, well. You don't have to eat it."*

Sometimes I'd feel myself getting annoyed or upset. After all, feeding my kids was *a lot* of work. I didn't need the complaints, thank you very much! But then, I'd pat myself on the back (literally) and tell myself I'd done my job. Voila! I'd stuck with our snack schedule, I chose a healthy, balanced snack for them, and I made it available. I was pleasant and calm. And I left it up to them to figure out what they were eating, how much, and how to settle themselves if they weren't entirely happy with the snack that day.

I tell you this because I know that snack time isn't always unicorns and rainbows. It can be a challenging time of feeding your kids. However, with a diplomatic approach, it can be easier. Your child will see you as a loving leader rather than a demanding authority figure, and you will be in control, not your child.

In Chapter Seven, you learned about monitoring and the difference between food restriction, or being a food cop, and an awareness of what your child's snacking patterns are throughout the day. In the last chapter, I discussed the role of feeding in appetite regulation, and how being tuned in to your child's cues helps you respond to his needs. This reinforces his ability to eat with intention and mindfulness. In this chapter, we're going even deeper into feeding. I'm uncovering what it means to use a diplomatic feeding style (a Love-with-Limits approach) and how to build your child's autonomy with snacking; and how to set up a responsive and flexible environment that encourages healthy choices and habits at snack time.

. . .

FEEDING STYLES, REVISITED

If you want to raise a *Smart Snacker*, you need to pay attention to how you're feeding him. I don't mean on a pretty plate and cut into cute shapes. I mean, what's your vibe? What's your approach?

Some parents don't think about or understand that the interaction with their children around food is laced with attitudes, belief systems, and intentions. For example, when I was a kid, my parents expected me to eat what they gave me. That expectation underlined every eating experience, from our daily meals to eating at relatives' homes and in restaurants. In my home, we did not waste food or insult the cook by not eating what was offered.

Researchers call these attitudes and intentions a feeding style. There are four different styles and most parents use one primarily, but there can be some mixing of styles too (Drayer, 2019).

Let's review them:

Controlling feeding style is known as a "parent-centered" approach to feeding. It emphasizes rules and expectations about eating, from trying new foods to completing a meal. Parents may pre-plate food for their children, use food rewards to motivate eating, or restrict certain foods to change their child's eating. Eating is directed by the parent rather than self-regulated by the child. Research suggests children are more likely to become resistant to trying new foods and are poor regulators of their eating. Weight problems, both underweight and overweight are correlated with this feeding style.

Indulgent feeding style is also known as an 'anything goes' style of feeding, reflecting a "child-directed" approach. The child is in charge rather than the parent in this scenario. For instance, even though the parent says no or sets a limitation, the child ultimately gets his way. Children of indulgent feeders may eat too many sweets and treats and may become overweight. This is because of few limits on calorie-dense foods.

Uninvolved feeding style may signify that feeding is a low priority for the parent. This may show up as irregular shopping, empty cabinets and refrigerators, and no plan for meals or snacks. Children who experience this feeding style may feel insecure about when they'll have their next meal, whether they'll like it and if it'll be enough. These kids may become overly focused on food and frequently question the details around snacks and mealtime.

Diplomatic feeding style is the love-with-limits approach, promoting independent thinking and self-regulation within the child, but also setting boundaries around food and eating. The diplomatic feeder determines the details around the snack or meal (what will be served, when it will happen, and where it will be served) and allows the child to decide whether he will eat what's prepared and how much. This is essentially the definition of Ellyn Satter's *Division of Responsibility in Feeding* and is a fundamental underpinning of positive feeding (Ellyn Satter Institute, 2016).

Let's review and repeat:

You:

- Decide about what will be served for snacks
- Decide where it will be eaten
- Determine what time your child gets it

Your child:

- Decides whether he will eat it

- Decides how much he will eat

Children who have parents with a diplomatic feeding style tend to be leaner, good at self-regulating their food consumption, and feel secure with food and eating. The most current research advocates this style of feeding as an effective approach for raising healthy kids.

So, what's your feeding style? Whatever it is, having self-awareness around your feeding style and your everyday actions is the first step to helping your child becoming a better snacker.

LOVE WITH LIMITS: THE GOLD STANDARD OF FEEDING

Perhaps you thought you were doing a good job with positive feeding, or maybe you could use some fine tuning. Wherever you are, I'm going to help you clearly understand the details of what it means to be diplomatic with feeding.

Why? All parents should move toward a diplomatic feeding style. Not only does it promote self-regulated eating, it lays the foundation of a positive relationship with food and promotes independent thinking and decision-making in children.

A diplomatic approach to feeding includes structure, boundaries, and guided choices. The good news? At this stage, you've learned a lot about diplomatic feeding because I've laced this book with the principles along the way. You learned about setting up a structure with snacks in Chapter One. In Chapter Five, you learned about boundaries. Now you'll learn about guided choices.

GUIDE YOUR CHILD'S CHOICES

. . .

In my experience, allowing kids to have a say, or a choice, results in better cooperation. I find when kids are respected and heard they are more willing to comply with the feeding structure. However, we can't give our kids complete control over food. One reason is because it overwhelms many kids to have open access and unlimited choices, and they may not make healthy decisions that serve them well. This is where guiding their choices can be helpful.

For young children, I suggest offering two food options. For example, at snack time you could offer hummus and pita chips or cereal and milk. Older kids can handle a few more options, but they can get overwhelmed too. Keep it contained and reasonable, such as peanut butter crackers, trail mix, or a mini cheese quesadilla. Outlining the options keeps you in charge of the food quality while allowing your child to make the choice without feeling overwhelmed.

BUILDING AUTONOMY WITH SNACKS

At the end of childhood, your goal is to have raised an autonomous human being. A child who knows how to feed herself, make healthy food choices, self-regulate her eating, and prepare food.

So how do you encourage your child to learn about nutrition and make good snack choices on her own? You encourage her autonomy. Promoting autonomy means you educate, involve, encourage, praise, reason, and negotiate with your child. Don't worry, this doesn't mean you are handing over your leadership!

But it means you weave these things into your daily feeding routines.

For example, involving your child in preparing snacks can be a powerful way to teach her about food, but also encourage fun and experimentation. Negotiating about what goes on the snack menu for the week gives your child a 'voice' in food decisions. This sends a message that you hear your child and will consider her ideas. How powerful this feedback is!

In negotiations around food, listening to your child's reasons and considering them is probably more important than your end decision. Educating about nutrition using natural opportunities such as baking together or shopping for food improves your child's ability to understand and allows her to decide using this knowledge.

I hope you can see the importance of building autonomy, as it is the backbone to your child's motivation, knowledge, and maturity with eating. So let's explore some practical ways you can build autonomy with snacking.

CREATIVE WAYS TO LET YOUR CHILD TAKE THE LEAD

One of the best ways to encourage autonomy is to let your child 'do' snacks on her own. Here are some ways to practice this:

MYO Snacks

MYO, or make your own, hands over the assembly of snacks to your child. I touched on this in Chapter Six and gave you some real food ideas to get going. As a reminder, if you're serving a peanut butter sandwich for a snack, you offer the knife (use a plastic one for young children), peanut butter, and bread, and let your child do the work. You can take this approach with quesadillas, cereal and milk, yogurt parfaits, trail mixes, and more. Put out the ingredients and let your child assemble them in the way she wants.

Set the Weekly Snack Menu

From picking out the general foods for snack time to determining which snack on which day, have your child help you plan the snack items for the week. You can take this a step further and have your child write out the grocery list for you.

Snack Drawers, Pantry Shelf, and a Refrigerator Section

Some parents have success with designating a snack drawer, pantry shelf, or refrigerator section that includes snacks for kids. At a determined time, allow kids to go there and pick their own snack. Of course, the quality of food in these locations is a consideration. I encourage you to choose nutritious options.

To conserve on costs, you can purchase some snacks in bulk, such as crackers, cereal, nuts, pretzels, and popcorn, and prepackage them into small plastic bags or reusable containers.

———

For the snack drawer or pantry shelf: Small bags of crackers; pretzels; pita chips; mini bagels; peanut butter cups; granola bars; nuts; trail mix; dry cereal boxes (or small bags); popcorn; fruit cups; applesauce cups; fruit and vegetable pouches; small chocolate milk cartons; seaweed snacks; veggie chips

. . .

For the refrigerator shelf: Yogurt cups, sticks, and smoothies; cheese blocks or sticks; small bags of baby carrots or other vegetables; hummus cups; cottage cheese cups; fruit cups; cream cheese cups

———

Encourage your child to mix and match. For instance, he might grab a mini bagel from the pantry and a cream cheese cup from the refrigerator, or pretzels from the pantry, and a hummus cup from the fridge. The combinations are endless!

I'll add a personal reflection: I tried this many years ago with my toddler and had a hard time controlling her wandering in and out of the kitchen all day long. Perhaps this would have worked better for us if she was older. As a result, I never tried it again, but I think it can work if you have kids who understand the 'kitchen is closed' boundary. (See Chapter Five for a refresher on this.)

If you find your kids are responding to this setup like Alyssa's kids did in Chapter One, reframe this approach. Perhaps this could be a tool for a day or for twice a week, rather than the standard way snacks are offered.

WHEN YOUR CHILD TRIES TO TAKE TOO MUCH CONTROL

It's inevitable that some kids will try to take advantage and push the limits around snacking. In my many years of working with families, parents have shared their fear of giving control to their child. They fear their kid would take over. Or that allowing some freedoms I'm suggesting would backfire and create more trouble. Let me explain this and offer some suggestions.

. . .

Your Child Helps Herself, Too Often

As I mentioned above, I had this same experience with my toddler. I decided it wasn't working for us and I shifted to scheduled snacks of my choosing and let her choose the "this or that" option. But what if your child is older and bolder?

A child who helps herself may try to tell you she wants more independence. I'd interpret it and call it out. You could say, *"It seems like you want more independence with snacking. Am I right?"* If she agrees, you can discuss some techniques I covered earlier. But, also reset the limits around eating in your home, such as the general timing for snacks, what to do if she's feeling hungry before snack time (e.g., ask you first), and reinforce a spirit of working together through problem solving and communication.

Your Child Refuses to Eat the Snack

Again, this often comes from wanting more independence or a voice, or it can stem from disliking what you're serving. If your child is being a rebel, ask her why. Try to get below the surface behavior and understand her motivations. If it's a desire for more independence, honor that and work through it.

If it's pushing your buttons, don't engage. Just state nicely, *"This is the snack for today. You don't have to eat it."* Sometimes kids just want to see if they can get their way with negative behavior. My advice is to stick with your plan and don't engage. Stay in charge.

If your child really doesn't like what you've offered, you can make a substitution or not. But try not to get into the routine of changing snack every day. Instead, invite your child to plan out the snack menu with you to avoid this scenario.

If you're a parent of a picky eater who snubs his nose at some of your snack offerings, hang in there. I know parents who try to expose their kids to new foods at snack time. They do this by offering a liked food with a new food. They don't sweat it if their child refuses to eat the new food, knowing that part of moving their picky eater forward is pushing the envelope a little. I think they are handling this situation well.

Your Child Is Sneaking Snacks

When parents come to me with concerns about sneaking food, they're often discouraged and embarrassed. For some parents, having a child who is sneaking food signifies problematic eating that can lead to health conditions. First, if this is your child, I want you to relax a bit. Many kids sneak food. Even mine have done this. Sometimes, they're just exercising their independence and taking food up to their rooms to eat without telling you.

What can you do? Sit down and have a chat with your child. Figure out why this behavior is happening. Is it hunger? Is it too much food restriction? Is it a desire to be in charge of snacking himself? One thing is certain, independent snacking will eventually surface as a reason, because as kids get older, they're developmentally driven to seek independence (hello, middle-schoolers and teenagers!). If this is the case, you must hand over more control to your child with parameters for her to follow. For example, my teens help themselves to their own snacks now. They know how to make a nutritious choice, and I trust them to eat snacks when they need them. However, they know we have a rule about eating on the first floor (no food in the bedrooms!) and they respect this, mostly.

If sneaking is related to hunger, recheck the nutritional quality of your snacks. Are they filling? Are they enough? Be sure, especially during a growth spurt, that snacks are growing with your child.

If food is too tightly controlled in your home, discuss this with your child. What feels right for her? And what feels right for you? Come to a compromise and work it out. Be clear about your food boundaries and make sure your child understands that you want her to feel satisfied with the food in your home.

NIBBLE ON THIS

As you can see, bringing a diplomatic feeding style to your snack table helps you stay in charge, while also encouraging food learning, autonomy, and healthy snacking. Remember, guiding your child with choices and supporting his autonomy development will go a long way to raising a *Smart Snacker*. Your child is growing and changing, and you must adapt alongside her. I'm confident you can do this!

Next, we'll explore your child's temperament in Chapter Ten: *T Is for Temperament*, because all these good practices cannot ignore the inherent personality and temperament your child possesses. Understanding this gives you powerful insight into what works for *your* child.

Take the Challenge!

Try one of my autonomy-building snack tips this week. Will you try a MYO snack, plan a snack menu for the week with your child, or designate a snack spot in your pantry, drawer, or fridge?

S N A C K S M A R T: T

T IS FOR TEMPERAMENT & DEVELOPMENT

W elcome to Chapter Ten: *T Is for Temperament &
Development*. Here, I'll explore what to expect
with your child's development and help you recognize temperament so you can see how it relates to his eating.
This understanding will help you have more empathy, patience,
and ultimately, confidence in how you respond to your child.
Because knowing who your child is and why he's behaving this
way is the insider's guide that can change your responses from
unproductive to positive.

Sometimes I feel like I've been through it all. With four
grown kids, I've navigated all the stages of child development
and learned the eating personalities and temperament they bring
to the table. Although I'm no child psychologist or developmental specialist, I recognize the value of understanding your
child's temperament and developmental stages. In fact, I think
this information is golden. It's incredibly powerful to understand
why your child is behaving the way he is and knowing he's not
doing it to irritate you.

At one time, one of my kids wanted to become a vegetarian.

Instead of being afraid of her motivations, I was curious to see how it would play out. Would she stick with it? Would she be open to learning how to be a healthy vegetarian? Would she eat beans, tofu, and vegetables? What did I need to teach her and tell her about being a healthy vegetarian? Could she be healthy? *Really?*

But then I put on my dietitian hat and remembered all the developmental stuff about teenagers. How teens are prone to impulsivity, experimentation, and a desire to be independent. I became calmer. And I waited it out. Ultimately, she reintroduced animal foods in her diet and reset the balance with a greater focus on plant foods.

I've seen similar scenarios play out with other parents over the years. The despair when a parent can't get their picky eater to try anything. The disappointment when a child shares fruit with a schoolmate as a trade for cookies. Or the fear when a teen starts a cleanse. These unsettling behaviors may leave parents feeling worried.

While I don't disregard the potential seriousness of these situations, I also recognize that there's a developmental, and potentially temperamental, backbone here. I want you to pinpoint this too. There is almost always a motivation behind behavior. Sometimes this motivation is simply related to *who* your child is and *where* he's at.

TODDLER TO TEEN: THE DEVELOPMENTAL ARC

Child development influences your child's eating. From toddler picky eating to adolescents seeking independence, children develop cognitively, socially, and emotionally along a continuum. They move through one stage, accomplish the developmental tasks, then move on to the next stage. We have age categories for each stage of development; however, children move through them not based on their age, but on their own timeline.

For example, we know that it's pretty common for toddlers between the ages of two and six to move through food neophobia, or the fear of new food. This makes them fussier about food, refusing foods they once liked, and stubborn about trying new foods. Many kids, however, don't move through picky eating by the age of six. For some, this stage will last longer. Likewise, teens want to make their own decisions. They may want to cook, choose their own snacks, or eat outside of the home, all to satisfy the urge to be independent. Again, completely normal.

While we know children move through these predictable phases as they grow into adulthood, they can confuse and frustrate parents. Yet, when you understand child development and all that it entails, it may make you a more empathetic parent who can see what is driving their behavior. Let's take a quick tour of what happens at each stage of childhood development. If you want to learn more about the infant, check out my book *The Smart Mom's Guide to Starting Solids*.

The Toddler

Toddlerhood is a complex time for parents. Your dependent baby is morphing into a little human who has a mind of his own. The theme of toddlerhood development is separation. Toddlers are experiencing a budding sense of independence. They're exploring the world around them with great interest, testing the limits, and understanding how to control themselves. Erik Erikson, a psychologist, describes toddlerhood as a time of struggle, during which toddlers are figuring out who they are as an individual and how to exert control over themselves and their world.

The feedback they receive from their environment helps them figure this out.

Physical growth slows down compared to the exponential growth in the first year of life. The toddler appetite shifts, fluctuating between voracious on some days and light or nonexistent on others. In a nutshell, toddlerhood is a time of picky eating for many families.

Combine the desire for independence and exploration with an unpredictable appetite, and it's no wonder toddlers and their eating cause their parents confusion, frustration, and worry.

Some typical eating behaviors during toddlerhood include:

- Refusing to eat foods previously liked
- Being afraid to try new foods (called neophobia)
- Wanting to eat certain foods or getting stuck on one food for a long period (called a food jag)
- Skipping meals or snacks

The good news? These behaviors are a natural and normal part of toddler development. They're expected. The bad news? If you're not prepared, they'll test your patience and may be the root of some of those negative feeding practices I mentioned in Chapter Nine. If you're struggling with feeding your toddler, my book *Try New Food: How to Help Picky Eaters Taste, Eat & Like New Foods* will help.

The Child

School-age children are at an interesting crossroads: They're learning at a fast pace and beginning to process more complex ideas. Yet, they see the world in absolutes (black or white, and right or wrong). They're also increasingly influenced by their peers, the media, and their community. For example, children want to be like their friends. If a friend has a new pair of jeans, or eats processed lunch packs at school, your child may ask you for the same. The drive for school-age children to be like their peers is strong.

Children are also susceptible to what they hear from authorities in their lives and from the media. Because they are black-and-white thinkers, they believe what they're told. This can play out with what they're exposed to from media outlets, such as TV, gaming, and the internet. It's hard for children to discern media intent from reality. For example, when healthy-appearing kids are portrayed eating junk food, kids may have difficulty understanding that too much junk food can negatively influence health. Or, they think it's cool to eat that way, not understanding the long-term implications.

During this time, your child's social-emotional development and his self-esteem is blooming. Erikson describes this as a time in life when children pursue *industry vs. inferiority*. It's the understanding through experiences that one is a capable human, or not. For example, if you still make your child's plate, he may get the message he's not able to do it himself. This can reinforce inferiority. Alternatively, if you allow your child to assemble his meals and snacks, you send the message you believe he's capable, reinforcing industry. *Industry vs. inferiority* plays out in all aspects of your child's life. On the sporting fields, in friendships, in school, and in your home.

Your child's sense of industry or inferiority is tied to his self-esteem development. A child who views himself as inferior, or "not capable," will struggle with confidence and self-esteem. Learning that one is skilled and good at something, or industrious, builds self-esteem.

As kids learn new skills, their self-esteem is nurtured. At home, getting them in the kitchen to cook and allowing them to make their own snacks are perfect opportunities to work on skill development and building self-esteem.

The Teen

Hold on to your hat. You're in for a ride! You may be prepped for typical teen rebellion: Driving too fast and staying out too late. But are you ready for food confusion, fad diets, and unhealthy eating? These fall into typical teenage development too. Why?

During adolescence, teens are thinking differently. The concrete thinking of children is changing to more sophisticated reasoning and judgement. The brain pathways are being refined, and this allows them to move toward abstract, long-term-consequence-type thinking and flexible problem solving. This is a good thing, but let me tell you, the process is rocky and rife with impulsivity, risk taking, and more separation. Teens value risk over reward. They're prone to risky decisions and behaviors. On the food front, they may experiment with food and eating behaviors like going vegan or using drastic diets to lose weight.

Adolescence is also a period of identity formation and separation from adult caretakers. In early adolescence, teens are less concerned with developing their own identity and more concerned with being part of a group. They're susceptible to peer pressure and outside influences, not unlike the child stage of development. This "psychology of belonging" allows young teens to identify with group norms and values. As teens get older, however, they become more self-assured and can make choices for themselves based on their values and individuality, rather than on group norms. They may reject following their group and branch out independently, embracing their self-identity.

· · ·

Navigating Child Development Well

During childhood, your child will move through these developmental stages. Some kids move through quickly, while others lag behind in a stage. How you interact and respond to your child related to this may influence how quickly (or how slowly) your child gets through each stage. I've seen parents unintentionally hold their kids back from developing as they should when they (the parents) are not ready for the stages and changes.

Picky eating, for instance, can drag on when parents interfere with their child's eating by helping their child eat or laying on the pressure. Helping your child too much as he interacts and experiences food may mean he's slow to learn and feel confident. And fighting for control of your teen's food decisions may mean you're embattled and at odds with one another, rather than nurturing your teen to care for himself.

Understanding your child's development and working with it, rather than against it, will always help your child move forward.

But child development isn't the end-all, be-all. There's another facet that deals with your child's personality: her temperament. Let's explore how this influences eating.

Your Child's Temperament and Eating Tendencies

How your child snacks and what he chooses is as much about personality, environment, and opportunity as it is about nutrition. Your child's temperament is a contributing force. It isn't always easy to see by watching your child eat, however. But when you tease out the facets of temperament, you can put the puzzle pieces together.

Here are some general aspects about temperament that give you some clues about your child:

Activity Level: What is your child's activity level? Does she wiggle around when trying to sit still? Get up from the table frequently? Or does she settle in for meals and snacks?

Regularity: Is your child regular about eating times, bowel movements, and sleeping times? Or is she irregular and unpredictable in these areas?

Adaptability: Is your child quick or slow to adapt to changes in her schedule? Or do changes cause a meltdown or a show of resistance?

Approach/Withdrawal: How does your child react to new people, new environments, or new foods? Does she engage and embrace or shy away and avoid?

Physical Sensitivity: How aware is your child of noises, temperature of food or environment, changes in taste, or the general "feel" of clothing?

Intensity of Reaction: How strong are your child's reactions? Is she energetic when laughing or crying or does she smile or fuss mildly?

Distractibility: Is your child easily distracted, or able to ignore distractions?

Positive or Negative Mood: How often does your child show joyful, pleasant behavior compared with fussy, unpleasant behavior?

Persistence: How long does your child continue with one activity? Does she persist if it's difficult?

As you can see, the traits of temperament vary, and the combinations are endless. It's most important to be aware of your child's tendencies and see if you can connect them with her eating. If she has an intense temperament, this may show up at the table through loud outbursts when you ask her to eat, or crying when she's upset. Or, you may have a child who gets up and down at the table (can't sit still), seems to be fussy at mealtime, or won't take no for an answer.

When I think about my own kids, I can easily see some temperament traits outlined above and how they expressed themselves in eating. For example, one of my kids was highly active, slow to adapt, bold with strangers, intense, and persistent. This is the child I referred to as "spirited." Her eating personality, though, was one of grazing and picking at meals. She could take food or leave it. She was generally too involved with other activities to pause and eat. Another child of mine was very regular in her eating, tended toward shyness and withdrawal from new people, mild in her responses, and one I considered timid, but an amiable child with which to live and feed. She was as regular with eating as they come.

Remember, with eating, your child brings his temperament to the table. You cannot change that, but you can adapt *your* responses and your environment to help her adapt better.

THREE KINDS OF EATERS

In my book, *Fearless Feeding: How to Raise Healthy Eaters from High Chair to High School*, my co-author and I identify three types of eaters to help parents understand their child's temperament and eating tendencies better. Which type of eater do you have?

The Eager Eater: These kids are adventurous and willing to try anything. They accept new foods easily and accumulate a variety of foods in their diet quickly. They may also have a big appetite.

The Somewhere-in-between Eater: This eater represents the vast majority of kids. They may be slow to warm up to new foods, but with repeated exposure and a positive atmosphere, they accept them.

The Cautious Eater: These are the timid eaters. They need time to check out new foods, get comfortable, and eventually add it to their food repertoire. These kids may be supertasters, have more sensory sensitivity, or be extremely picky.

Knowing the eater you have, whether cautious, eager, or in-between, helps you understand her reactions and where she's coming from.

THE SNACKER PROFILE: COMMON SCENARIOS AND HOW TO MANAGE THEM

Over the years, I've found common themes around snacking habits. Here, I want to further identify some of these behaviors, tie them to child development and temperament, and provide some suggestions for managing them.

The Starving-after-School Kid

Your child enters the car or your home, *starving*. How could she be this hungry?

Here, you'll want to rewind the day and look at her *actual* intake earlier in the day. You may see it was mediocre. You may have evidence to support your case: leftovers in the lunchbox or a half-eaten bowl of cereal in the morning. When kids eat inadequately at the beginning and middle of the day, they may be starving when they return home.

Why does this happen? Your child may be very social at lunchtime and not eat enough. She may feel timid about eating in front of others, preferring to eat at home. Or, she may not like what you packed for lunch.

Remedy: Of course, we want kids to eat at school, but sometimes there are reasons for not eating that have nothing to do with food. While you'll want to encourage your child to eat a hearty breakfast and lunch, you'll also want to talk with your child and explore other reasons. If distraction is the cause, emphasize eating the main entrée so that your child gets a wider variety of nutrients to sustain her appetite until she comes home. If timidness is the reason, coach your child through the lunch scene and help her find reasonable ways to eat. Get your child's input on satisfying lunches and work together toward a solution.

The Never-Full Kid

Within an hour after a meal, this child is hungry and asking for more food.

Why does this happen? Several reasons may contribute to this scenario, such as not eating enough food at mealtime, not being satisfied with what was served and eaten, eating the wrong foods (nutrient-poor foods), a habit of asking, or physical hunger related to a growth spurt. Head hunger, boredom, or emotions can also be the culprit, as can your child's eating style of grazing throughout the day.

Remedy: Get back on a regular schedule (3 meals + 1–3 snacks depending on your child's age). Reassess the nutrition your child is getting and boost the balance of food and nutrients, erring on the side of wholesome and nutritious. Close the kitchen between meals and snacks and encourage your child to do other activities. If it's head hunger, chat about the difference between physical hunger and head hunger and help your child discern between the two. (Refer to Chapter Nine for more on hunger.)

The Take-It-or-Leave-It Kid

This child never seems very interested in eating.

Why does this happen? Some kids aren't big on snacking. I know, I have one. She'd rather have three square meals and not deal with snacks. The take-it-or-leave-it kid may also be called a "grazer," nibbling through the day and saving his appetite for meals. This is related to your child's temperament.

Remedy: There are no big changes you need to make here. It's more about accepting this eating style and taking on the role of snack *provider*. Stay on a schedule with snacks and let your child know there is something planned and available. If she refuses, don't sweat it. Move onto the next meal or snack, and make sure it's wholesome, nutritious, balanced, and satisfying. Above all, let your child self-regulate his appetite.

The Junk Food Junkie

This child loves ultra-processed foods, sweets, and fried foods. Parents sometimes say, "He won't eat anything unless it's junk!"

Why does this happen? Ultra-processed foods are tasty, which will almost always get a child's attention and favor. But kids are also influenced by what other kids eat, and they often request the same foods. This is developmentally normal. The regular presence of these foods in the home or a child's environment will make it difficult to change this eating habit. Check yourself: Are you purchasing these foods regularly? Is your child regularly exposed to junk food outside of your home?

Remedy: Contrary to popular belief, you *can* reprogram this situation. Make sure your child is getting exposed to plenty of nutritious foods and you are being a role model for eating them. Use and teach your child about the 90–10 Rule (Go to Chapter Two to revisit this if you need to). You'll negotiate a happy middle ground, one that allows Fun Foods, but sets a limit. Set a family mantra or policy about eating indulgent foods like sweets, treats, and junk food. Kids have an easier time navigating these foods when they have a response they can use like, "*My family likes these foods, but we don't eat them every day.*"

NIBBLE ON THIS

As you can see, understanding your child's development and temperament gives you a new frame for interpreting what's going on with her snacking. Remember, you cannot change your child's stage of development, or her inherent temperament. You must work with it.

Take the Challenge!

Take some time to acknowledge your child's temperament. Who is she as an eater? Assess where she's at in her development. How can you parent better? Do you need to stop helping your child eat? Give her more freedom in the kitchen? Trust she can decide about her diet or support her food journey? Try to alter your response to your child based on this new awareness.

RAISING A SMART SNACKER THE SMART MOM WAY

Congratulations! You've reached the end of this book and you've learned a lot! Sure, giving your child healthy food is part of raising a *Smart Snacker*; however, as you've learned, there's more to it.

If you feel completely off track with snacking in your home, that's okay. You can make things better by starting with "S" in Chapter One. Move on to the next letter when you're ready.

If you get frustrated or stuck in a rut with snacks, or you detect your child is falling into unhealthy snacking habits, you'll need to troubleshoot. Maybe you need to tighten up your snacking routine. Perhaps you need to spice things up with fresh snack options. Or maybe your child is changing and you need to change too. Whatever is going on, you can find solutions. Use the SNACK SMART acronym to help you.

Let's recap what it means to SNACK SMART.

S Is for Snacking Intervals

Set up a schedule and routine around the timing of snacks.

This routine will become rhythmic and flow naturally. It will support your child's appetite cues and help him recognize those internal signals for eating.

Remember, young children need more snacks than older kids. Based on your child's age and your family's day-to-day schedule, map out the times for daily snacks. If things get wonky because of schedules, school, work, or other obligations, rework your timing and routine so it's consistent from day to day.

N Is for Nutrient-Rich Foods, Most of the Time

Real, wholesome food is your friend when you're targeting healthy snacks that provide a boost of nutrients to your child, especially with nutrients that are missing or have low amounts in the diets of many kids. Bring variety to the snack table and rotate foods within food groups to spark interest and better nutrition.

It's okay to work in sweets and treats, but the lion's share of options should focus on nutrient-rich foods. Don't let *Fun Foods* crowd out nutritious snacks. Create the best of both worlds: Use the Fun Food + a nutrient-rich food strategy (e.g., chocolate chip cookies and milk) when treats are the snacking option.

A Is for Amounts Matter

Snacks are mini meals. Small bites. A nibble or nosh. Size-able portions can turn a snack into a meal, which defeats your meal-and-snack structure. Serve the portions that align with your child's age as a starting point. Then, let your child's appetite provide guidance for second helpings.

As kids grow, they will be hungrier, and because they love snacks, they may want more. An additional piece of fruit to the snack can cover this extra hunger (or offer more veggies, milk, or other nutritious item). The point of starter portions is to help you tune in to your child's appetite and support it, rather than giving more food and potentially turning that snack into a meal.

C Is for Calories Count

Snacks contribute to your child's overall caloric intake and this can be a help or a drag on her health. If your eye is on calories all the time (and controlling or limiting them), you may miss the secret weapon to satisfaction. Remember, quality calories, and the filling nutrients of protein, fiber, and fat will help your child feel satisfied after eating.

If you're on the go, in a pinch, or just lacking inspiration, it's okay to use packaged snacks or even calorie-controlled snacks, but work in some protein, fiber, or fat. This will take the satisfaction factor up a notch.

K Is for Keep it Contained

Boundaries, boundaries, boundaries! Kids do well when they know the rules and have the family food system and routines identified. These help your child know what to do and how to behave when you're not around. And they help you successfully keep snacks in their place. Whether you put in place a "kitchen is closed," "no food in front of the TV," or other boundary, get clear on the ones you want to maintain in your home.

For example, figure out where you want snacking to occur, and where you don't. Be clear about this with your child. If snacking gets too loose, rein it in by re-establishing the boundaries. This will be one of your best defenses against poor food choices and overeating.

S Is for Simple & Easy

Let's get rid of the "Pin-worthy" snack. Keep snacks interesting and fun by creating tasty, easy, food options. Whether it be healthy homemade snacks, cute plate faces or a Make-Your-Own snack platter, the goal here is to make snacks simple, easy, and enticing for your child.

If you're in a snack rut, or lack inspiration, come back to this chapter and the Appendix for creative (and easy) snack ideas!

M Is for Monitor & Model Eating

Being a good food monitor means you're aware of what your child is eating and you adjust your food plan as needed. That means you don't have to freak out if your child has eaten too many sweets. You can adjust the menu, take a break for a day or two, or take sweets in stride and regroup the following week.

Monitoring your child's eating can promote healthy snacking. Be careful, however. It can backfire, turning you into a food cop who is too restrictive and creating more eating problems. Revisit Chapter Seven if you need help with language and responses to challenging snacking situations.

The goal is to be an excellent role model of health for your child and keep track of his eating, both of which enable you to better guide your child to be a *Smart Snacker*.

A Is for Appetite Awareness

One of the most important skills you can teach your child is to be tuned in to his body, especially his appetite signals. A keen sense of hunger, satisfaction, and fullness will help your child be better at regulating his eating.

Is your child is overeating? Dig into why. Is she truly hungry? Or does she "think" she's hungry? Tease this out, as it can be the underlying reason for extra snacking. Reinforce your snack schedule and eating boundaries. Keep filling nutrients front and center so you can stay ahead of hunger. Structure and smart food choices can be your ally as you retrain your child's snacking habits and help her eat with mindfulness.

R Is for Responsive & Flexible

You can't become a *Smart Mom* without understanding feeding kids and the power you possess when you get this right. Using a love-with-limits feeding approach keeps you in charge, but encourages your child's autonomy and independence.

If your child is sneaking snacks or refusing them, perhaps he needs more autonomy. Although this may seem counterproductive, providing guidance around food choices and letting your child take the lead with snacks is the fast path to cooperation and independent, healthy snacking. You can do this no matter your child's age!

T Is for Temperament & Development

Your kid is who he is. And he's where he's at. His temperament and developmental stage will always influence his motivations, desires, and behaviors around food and eating. Having a good understanding on this is fundamental. Although you cannot change your child's inherent temperament or his developmental stage, you can learn to work with it.

If you're at a loss for understanding what's going on with your child, examine his characteristics and where he's at along the developmental arc. Is he going through a food jag? Is he mimicking his friend group? Is he experimenting? Unlock your understanding of the behaviors or choices you're seeing and your responses and interactions will be more effective.

. . .

You Are a *Smart Mom!*

There's no doubt in my mind you're now equipped with the knowledge you need, along with some inspiration, to be a *Smart Mom* who raises a *Smart Snacker*.

One who knows which foods to offer for snack, how to promote eating snacks to satisfy appetite, cravings, and enjoyment, and who can be flexible with sweets and treats, balancing them in the overall diet.

As we part ways, I want to remind you of a few more things:

Your child's snacking habits do not define you as a good parent or bad parent. Remember, your child is learning about food, his appetite, food preferences, and more. Things will change.

Put your best foot forward by setting up a food environment that encourages healthy snacking, be a force of positive feeding, and understand your child's developmental stage and temperament. These are your secret weapons.

Don't let others' standards define your feeding approach or food options. You get to raise your children the way you want.

Not only are you a feeder, you're a teacher and a guide. Help your child learn about food, his body and appetite, and the power of outside forces so he grows in his autonomy and independence with snacking.

My hope for you is that healthy snacking becomes a piece of cake for you and yours. That you learn to love this part of eating because you understand the role it plays in your child's diet. If you get frustrated, worried, or discouraged, go back to the SNACK SMART acronym and revisit the principles. It'll help you uncover the root of your challenge and set you back on the right track.

Above all, enjoy snacking with your child!

WANT MORE FROM JILL?

If you'd like more help on your journey of feeding and raising your child, the following resources will help:

1.) Grab My Free "Nourish a Healthy Child" Checklist
This framework and checklist gives you the big overview of what it takes to nourish your child, inside and out. Go to www. jillcastle.com/ and enter your details.

2.) Listen to The Nourished Child Podcast
Join me every other Thursday for The Nourished Child podcast where I interview experts and professionals about child nutrition, feeding kids and dealing with the ups and downs of raising healthy ones.
www.jillcastle.com/podcast

3.) Check out My Books for Parents
I have several guidebooks and print books, available on my parent education website, TheNourishedChild.com.

- Fuel Up! 35+ Dinner Recipes for Young Athletes
- 25+ Fast & Nutritious Breakfasts for Young Athletes
- The Essential Nutrients for Kids
- The Healthy Snack Planner for Kids
- The Calcium Handbook
- Try New Food: Help Picky Eaters Taste, Eat & Like New Foods
- Eat Like a Champion: Performance Nutrition for Your Young Athlete
- Fearless Feeding: How to Raise Healthy Eaters from High Chair to High School (2nd Edition)

4.) Check out my Classes and Workshops on The Nourished Child

Take your learning even deeper with my comprehensive courses for parents and caretakers, including:

- The Nourished Child Blueprint
- The ADHD Diet for Kids
- Eat Like a Champion
- Eat in Peace workshop

REVIEW MY BOOK

Would you take a minute to review this book?

It would mean so much to me!

Reviews help me get better at writing. They also motivate me to keep going and creating relevant and useful books for readers like you.

You can rate and write a review where ever you bought this book.

REFERENCES

Introduction

Centers for Disease Control. (2018). *Obesity.* https://www.cdc.gov/healthyschools/obesity/index.htm

Smith, L.P., Ng S.W., & Popkin B.M (2013). Trends in US home food preparation and consumption: Analysis of national nutrition surveys and time use studies from 1965–1966 to 2007–2008. *Nutrition Journal,* 12, 45.

Devenyns, J. (2019, November 11). 59% of adults prefer snacking to meals, Mondelez study finds. *Food Dive.* https://www.fooddive.com/news/59-of-adults-prefer-snacking-to-meals-mondelez-study-finds/567006/

Shriver, L.H., Marriage, B.J., Bloch, T.D., Spees, C.K., Ramsay, S.A., Watowicz R.P., & Taylor, C.A. (2017). Contribution of snacks to dietary intakes of young children in the United States. *Maternal & Child Nutrition,* 14(1): e12454.

Health Aff (Millwood) (2010). *Trends in Snacking among US Children*. 29(3), 398–404. https://www.ncbi.nlm.nih.gov/pmc/articles/PMC2837536/#__ffn_sectitle

Watson, E. (2013). Continuous snacking: US kids eat 4.1 snacks a day, while teens eat 3.8 snacks a day, says NPD Group. *Food Navigator-USA*. https://www.foodnavigator-usa.com/Article/2013/09/10/Continuous-snacking-US-kids-eat-4.1-snacks-a-day-while-teens-eat-3.8-snacks-a-day-says-NPD-Group#

Topper, A. (2015). A snacking nation: 94% of Americans snack daily. *Mintel*. https://www.mintel.com/press-centre/food-and-drink/a-snacking-nation-94-of-americans-snack-daily

Grand View Research (2019). *Healthy Snacks Market Size, Share & Trends Analysis Report by Product (Dried fruit, Cereal & Granola Bars, Nuts & Seeds, Meat, Trail Mix), By Region, Vendor Landscape, and Segment Forecasts, 2019-2025*. https://www.grandviewresearch.com/industry-analysis/healthy-snack-market

Moss, M. (2013, February 20).The extraordinary science of addictive junk food. *The New York Times Magazine*. https://www.nytimes.com/2013/02/24/magazine/the-extraordinary-science-of-junk-food.html

---

Chapter One

KidsHealth from Nemours (n.d.). *Your digestive system*. https://kidshealth.org/en/kids/digestive-system.html

American Academy of Pediatrics (n.d.). *Toddler – Food and Feeding*. https://www.aap.org/en-us/advocacy-and-policy/aap-health-initiatives/HALF-Implementation-Guide/Age-Specific-Content/Pages/Toddler-Food-and-Feeding.aspx

Shield, J.E. (2019). *When should my kids snack?* Kids Eat Right from the Academy of Nutrition and Dietetics. https://www.eatright.org/food/nutrition/dietary-guidelines-and-myplate/when-should-my-kids-snack

------

Chapter Two

Dietary Guidelines Advisory Committee (2020). *Scientific Report of the 2020 Dietary Guidelines Advisory Committee: Advisory Report to the Secretary of Agriculture and the Secretary of Health and Human Services.* U.S. Department of Agriculture, Agricultural Research Service, Washington, DC.

U.S. Department of Agriculture, Agricultural Research Service. (2016). *Nutrient Intakes from Food and Beverages: Mean Amounts Consumed per Individual, by Gender and Age,* What We Eat in America, NHANES 2013–2014.

Office of Dietary Supplements (2020). *Vitamin D. Fact Sheet for Health Professionals.* U.S. Department of Health and Human Services, National Institutes of Health. https://ods.od.nih.gov/factsheets/VitaminD-HealthProfessional/

Georgieff, M.K. (2017). Iron assessment to protect the developing brain, *The American Journal of Clinical Nutrition,* 106 (Supplement 6), 1588S–1593S.

https://doi.org/10.3945/ajcn.117.155846

Office of Dietary Supplements (2020). *Vitamin E. Fact Sheet for Health Professionals*. U.S. Department of Health and Human Services, National Institutes of Health. https://ods.od.nih.gov/factsheets/VitaminE-HealthProfessional/

Office of Dietary Supplements (2020). *Omega-3 Fatty Acids. Fact Sheet for Health Professionals*. U.S. Department of Health and Human Services, National Institutes of Health. https://ods.od.nih.gov/factsheets/Omega3FattyAcids-HealthProfessional/

ChooseMyPlate (2020). Center for Nutrition Policy and Promotion, U.S. Department of Agriculture. https://www.choosemyplate.gov/

Neelakantan, N., Seah, J.Y.H., van Dam, R. M. (2020). The effect of coconut oil consumption on cardiovascular risk factors. *Circulation*. 141, 803-814.

————

Chapter Three

Steenhuis, I.H., Leeuwis, F.H., Vermeer, W.M. (2010). Small, medium, large or supersize: trends in food portion sizes in The Netherlands. *Public Health Nutrition*. 13(6), 852-7.

Hetherington, M.M. & Blundell-Birtill, P. (2018). The portion size effect and overconsumption–towards downsizing solutions for children and adolescents. *Nutrition Bulletin*. 43, 61-68.

ChooseMyPlate (2020). Center for Nutrition Policy and Promotion, U.S. Department of Agriculture. https://www.choosemyplate.gov/

Food & Drug Administration (2020). *The New Nutrition Facts Label*. www.fda.gov/NewNutritionFactsLabel

—————

Chapter Four

Mozaffarian, D., Tao Hao, P.H., Rimm, E. B., Willett, W.C., & Hu, F.B. (2011). Changes in diet and lifestyle and long-term weight gain in women and men. *New England Journal of Medicine*. 364, 2392–2404.

British Nutrition Foundation. (2020, October 10). *The Quality Calorie (QC) Concept*. https://www.nutrition.org.uk/healthyliving/helpingyoueatwell/qualitycalorie

Chambers, L., McCrickerd, K., & Yeomans, M. R. (2015). Optimising foods for satiety. *Trends in Food Science & Technology*. 41, 149-160.

Westerterp K. R. (2004). Diet induced thermogenesis. *Nutrition & Metabolism*. 1, 5.

Arguin, H., Tremblay, A., Blundell, J. E., Depres, J-P., Richard, D., Lamarche, B. & Drapeau, V. (2017). Impact of a non-restrictive satiating diet on anthropometrics, satiety responsiveness and eating behaviour traits in obese men displaying a high or a low satiety phenotype. *British Journal of Nutrition*. 118, 750-760.

Kerr, J.A., Jansen, P.W., Mensah, F.K. Gibbons, K., Olds, T. S., Clifford, J. A., Burgner, D., Gold, L., Baur, L. A., & Wake, M. (2019). Child and adult snack food intake in response to manipulated pre-packaged snack item quantity/variety and snack box size: a population-based randomized trial. *International Journal of Obesity.* 43, 1891–1902.

Bailey, R. L., Fulgoni, V. L., & Gaine, P. C. (2018). Sources of added sugars in young children, adolescents, and adults with low and high intakes of added sugars. *Nutrients.* 10, 102.

American Heart Association. (2016, August). *Kids and added sugars: How much is too much?* https://www.heart.org/en/news/2018/05/01/kids-and-added-sugars-how-much-is-too-much

Dietary Guidelines Advisory Committee (2020). *Scientific Report of the 2020 Dietary Guidelines Advisory Committee: Advisory Report to the Secretary of Agriculture and the Secretary of Health and Human Services.* U.S. Department of Agriculture, Agricultural Research Service, Washington, DC.

———

Chapter Five

Nelson, J. B. (2017). Mindful eating: The art of presence while you eat. *Diabetes Spectrum.* 30, 171-174.

Yee, A. Z., Lwin, M. O., Ho, S. S. (2017). The influence of parental practices on child promotive and preventive food consumption behaviors: a systematic review and meta-analysis.

International Journal of Behavior, Nutrition & Physical Activity. 14(1), 47.

Peck, T., Scharf, R. J., Conaway, M. R., DeBoer, M. D. (2015). Viewing as little as 1 hour of TV daily is associated with higher change in BMI between kindergarten and first grade. *Obesity* (Silver Spring). 23,1680-1686.

Liang, J., Matheson, B. E., & Boutelle, K. N. (2016). Parental control and overconsumption of snack foods in overweight and obese children. *Appetite.* 100, 181-188.

———

Chapter Six

Christnacht, C. & Sullivan B. (2020, May 8). *About two-thirds of the 23.5 million working women with children under 18 worked full-time in 2018.* Retrieved September 2, 2020, from https://www.census.gov/library/stories/2020/05/the-choices-working-mothers-make.html

Geiger, A. W., Livingston, G. & Bialik, K. (2019, May 8). *6 Facts about US Moms.* Retrieved September 2, 2020 from https://www.pewresearch.org/fact-tank/2019/05/08/facts-about-u-s-mothers/.

Livingston, G. (2018, September 24). *Stay-at-home moms and dads account for about one-in-five US parents.* Retrieved September 2, 2020 from https://www.pewresearch.org/fact-tank/2018/09/24/stay-at-home-moms-and-dads-account-for-about-one-in-five-u-s-parents/

Coulthard, H. & Sealy, A. (2017) Play with your food! Sensory play is associated with tasting of fruits and vegetables in preschool children. *Appetite.* 113, 84-90.

———

Chapter Seven

Savage, J. S., Fisher, J. O., & Birch, L. L. (2007). Parental influence on eating behavior. *Journal of Law, Medicine & Ethics.* 35, 22-34.

Scaglioni, S., De Cosmi, V. & Agostini, C. (2018). Factors influencing children's eating behaviours. *Nutrients.* 10, 706.

Vaughn, A. E., Ward, D. S., & Power, T. G. (2016). Fundamental constructs in food parenting practices: a content map to guide future research. *Nutrition Reviews.* 74, 98-117.

Blaine, R. E., Kachurak, A., Davison, K. K., Klabunde, R., & Fisher, J. O. (2017). Food parenting and child snacking: a systematic review. *The International Journal of Behavioral Nutrition and Physical Activity.* 14, 146.

Liang, J., Matheson, B. E., & Boutelle, K. N. (2016). Parental control and overconsumption of snack foods in overweight and obese children. *Appetite.* 100, 181-188.

2009 study international journal of behavioural nutrition and physical activity short order cooking

Johnson, S. L. (2016). Developmental and environmental influences on young children's vegetable preferences and consumption. *Advances in Nutrition*. 7, 220S-231S.

Ellis, J. M., Galloway, A. T., Webb, R. M., Martz, D. M., & Farrow, C. V. (2016). Recollections of pressure to eat during childhood, but not picky eating, predict young adult eating behavior. *Appetite*. 97, 58-63.

DeCosta, P., Moller P., Frost, M. B., & Olsen A. (2017). Changing children's eating behaviour–A review of experimental research. 113, 327-357.

Galindo, L., Power, T. G., & Hughes, S. O. Predicting preschool children's eating in the absence of hunger from maternal pressure to eat: A longitudinal study of low-income, Latina mothers. (2018). *Appetite*. 120, 281-286.

Galloway, A. T., Fiorito, L. M., & Birch, L. L. (2006). 'Finish your soup.' *Appetite*. 46, 318-323.

Jansen, P. W., de Barse, L.M., & Tiemeier, H. (2017). Bi-directional associations between child fussy eating and parents' pressure to eat: who influences whom? *Physiology & Behavior*. 176, 101–106.

Houldcroft, L., Farrow, C., & Haycraft, E. (2014). Perceptions of parental pressure to eat and eating behaviours in preadolescents: the mediating role of anxiety. *Appetite*. 80, 61–69.

––––––

Chapter Eight

Lansigan, R. K., Emond, J. A., & Gilbert-Diamond, D. (2015). Understanding eating in the absence of hunger among young children: A systematic review of existing studies. *Appetite*. 0, 36–47.

———

Chapter Nine

Drayer, L. (2018, October 4). *Of the four parental 'feeding styles,' only one is good for kids' health, experts say.* CNN. https://www.cnn.com/2018/10/04/health/parenting-food-drayer/index.html

Ellyn Satter Institute (2016). *Ellyn Satter's Division of Responsibility in Feeding.* https://www.ellynsatterinstitute.org/wp-content/uploads/2016/11/handout-dor-tasks-cap-2016.pdf

———

Chapter Ten

Erikson, E. H. (1950). Childhood and Society. New York: Norton.

Castle, J. L. & Jacobsen, M. T. (2019). Fearless Feeding: How to Raise Healthy Eaters from High Chair to High School. Fearless Feeding Press.

———

Appendix

Haytowitz, D. B., Ahuja, J. K.C., Wu, X., Somanchi, M., Nickle, M., Nguyen, Q. A., Roseland, J. M., Williams, J. R., Patterson, K. Y., Li, Y., & Pehrsson, P. R. (2019). USDA National Nutrient Database for Standard Reference, Legacy Release. Nutrient Data Laboratory, Beltsville Human Nutrition Research Center, ARS, USDA. https://data.nal.usda.gov/dataset/usda-national-nutrient-database-standard-reference-legacy-release. Accessed 2020-10-31.

ACKNOWLEDGMENTS

This book wouldn't be possible without the support of my family, friends and colleagues. Special thanks goes out to Maryann Jacobsen for her direction and my self-publishing mastermind crew who keep me on task.

Thanks to Arnetta Jackson for her editing and proof-reading skills. Jen Henning for her masterful book cover design. And to my readers, especially Team Smart Mom for providing valuable feedback.

ABOUT THE AUTHOR

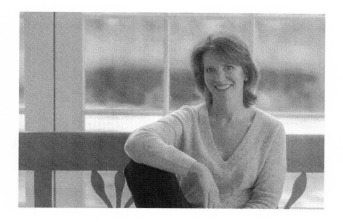

Jill Castle has practiced as a registered dietitian/nutritionist in the field of pediatric nutrition for three decades. Formerly a clinical pediatric dietitian at Massachusetts General Hospital and Children's Hospital, Boston, and a childhood nutrition private practice owner, Jill currently works as an author, online educator, consultant, and speaker.

She is the author of several books and is the founder of The Nourished Child, an educational website for parents who want to learn more about child nutrition and feeding their kids. She's also the voice behind The Nourished Child podcast.

Jill has been published in peer-reviewed journals, textbooks, consumer books, cookbooks, websites, and other blogs. She is a national and international speaker, focused on topics related to childhood nutrition and feeding kids of all ages.

She's regularly quoted in popular print and online publications as a leading childhood nutrition expert.

She lives in Connecticut with her husband and family. For more about Jill, go to www.JillCastle.com.

APPENDIX

Appendix A: Food Sources of Selected Nutrients

(Highest down to Lowest Amounts)

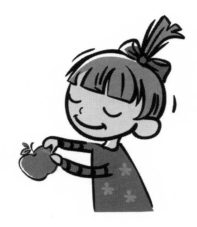

Appendix A.1: Iron-Rich Foods

Food Sources (Portion Size): Iron content

Heme Iron

Chicken liver, pan-fried (3 ounces): 11 mg
Oysters, canned (3 ounces): 5.7 mg
Beef liver, pan-fried (3 ounces): 5.2 mg
Beef, chuck, blade roast, braised (3 ounces): 3.1 mg
Turkey, dark meat, roasted (3 ounces): 2 mg
Beef, ground, 85% lean, broiled (3 ounces): 2.2 mg
Beef, top sirloin, steak, broiled (3 ounces): 1.6 mg
Tuna, light, canned in water (3 ounces): 1.3 mg
Turkey, light meat, roasted (3 ounces): 1.1 mg
Chicken, dark meat, roasted (3 ounces): 1.1 mg
Chicken, light meat, roasted (3 ounces): 0.9 mg
Tuna, fresh, yellowfin, cooked (3 ounces): 0.8 mg
Crab, Alaskan king, cooked (3 ounces): 0.7 mg
Pork, loin chop, broiled (3 ounces): 0.7 mg
Shrimp, mixed species, cooked (4 large): 0.3 mg
Halibut, cooked (3 ounces): 0.2 mg

Non-heme Iron

Cold cereal, 100% iron fortified (3/4 cup): 18 mg

Oatmeal, prepared with water (1 packet): 11 mg

Soybeans, boiled (1 cup): 8.8 mg

Lentils, boiled (1 cup): 6.6 mg

Beans, kidney, boiled (1 cup): 5.2 mg

Beans, lima, large, boiled (1 cup): 4.5 mg

Cold cereal, 25% iron fortified (3/4 cup): 4.5 mg

Blackeye peas, boiled (1 cup): 4.3 mg

Beans, navy, boiled (1 cup): 4.3 mg

Beans, black, boiled (1 cup): 3.6 mg

Beans, pinto, boiled (1 cup): 3.6 mg

Tofu, raw, firm (1/2 cup): 3.4 mg

Spinach, fresh, boiled (1/2 cup): 3.2 mg

Spinach, canned (1/2 cup): 2.5 mg

Spinach, frozen (1/2 cup): 1.9 mg

Raisins, seedless, packed (1/2 cup): 1.6 mg

Grits, white, enriched (1 cup): 1.5 mg

Molasses (1 tablespoon): 0.9 mg

Bread, white (1 slice): 0.9 mg

Bread, whole-wheat (1 slice) : 0.7 mg

Appendix A.2: Zinc-Rich Foods

Food (Portion Size): Zinc content

Oysters, breaded & fried (3 ounces): 493 mg

Beef chuck roast, braised (3 ounces): 47 mg

Crab, Alaska king, cooked (3 ounces): 43 mg

Beef patty, broiled (3 ounces): 35 mg

Breakfast cereal, 25% DV for zinc (3/4 cup): 25 mg

Lobster, cooked (3 ounces): 23 mg

Pork chop, loin, cooked (3 ounces): 19 mg

Baked beans, canned (1/2 cup): 19 mg

Chicken, dark meat, cooked (3 ounces): 16 mg

Yogurt, fruit, low fat (8 ounces): 11 mg

Cashews, dry roasted (1 ounce): 11 mg

Chickpeas, cooked (1/2 cup): 9 mg

Cheese, Swiss (1 ounce): 8 mg

Oatmeal, instant (1 packet): 7 mg

Milk, low-fat or nonfat (1 cup): 7 mg

Almonds, dry roasted (1 ounce): 6 mg

Kidney beans, cooked (1/2 cup): 6 mg

Chicken breast, roasted (1/2 breast): 6 mg

Cheese, cheddar or mozzarella (1 ounce): 6 mg

Peas, green, frozen, cooked (1/2 cup): 3 mg

Flounder or sole, cooked (3 ounces): 2 mg

Appendix A.3: Vitamin C-Rich Foods

Food (Portion Size): Vitamin C content

Red pepper, sweet, raw (1/2 cup): 158 mg
Orange juice (3/4 cup): 155 mg
Orange (1 medium): 117 mg
Grapefruit juice (3/4 cup): 117 mg
Kiwifruit (1 medium): 107 mg
Green pepper, sweet, raw (1/2 cup): 100 mg
Broccoli, cooked (1/2 cup): 85 mg
Strawberries, fresh, sliced (1/2 cup): 82 mg
Brussels sprouts, cooked (1/2 cup): 80 mg
Vegetable juice cocktail (1 cup): 67 mg
Grapefruit (1/2 medium): 65 mg
Broccoli, raw (1/2 cup): 65 mg
Ready-to-eat cereals (3/4 - 1 1/3 cup): 60-61 mg
Tomato juice (3/4 cup): 55 mg
Cantaloupe (1/2 cup): 48 mg
Cabbage, cooked (1/2 cup): 47 mg
Papaya (1/2 cup): 43 mg
Cauliflower, raw (1/2 cup): 43 mg
Pineapple (1/2 cup): 39 mg
Potato, baked (1 medium): 28 mg
Tomato, raw (1 medium): 28 mg
Kale, cooked from fresh (1/2 cup): 27 mg
Tangerine (1 medium): 24 mg
Mango (1/2 cup): 23 mg
Spinach, cooked (1/2 cup): 15 mg
Green peas, frozen, cooked (1/2 cup): 13 mg

Appendix A.4: Calcium-Rich Food Sources

Food (Portion Size): Calcium content

Plain yogurt, nonfat (8 ounces): 452 mg
Romano cheese (1 1/2 ounces): 452 mg
Yogurt, fruit, low fat (8 ounces): 338–384 mg
Ricotta cheese, part skim (1/2 cup): 337 mg
Mozzarella, part skim (1.5 ounces): 333 mg
Sardines, canned in oil, with bones (3 ounces): 325 mg
Cheddar cheese (1.5 ounces): 307 mg
Low-fat milk (1%) (1 cup): 305 mg
Orange juice, calcium fortified (1 cup): 300 mg
Nonfat milk (8 ounces): 299 mg
Reduced-fat milk (2%) (8 ounces): 293 mg
Low-fat chocolate milk (1%) (1 cup): 290 mg
Buttermilk (8 ounces): 282–350 mg
Whole milk (8 ounces): 276 mg
Reduced fat (2%) chocolate milk (1 cup): 272 mg
Tofu, firm with calcium sulfate* (1/2 cup): 253 mg
Salmon, pink, canned (3 ounces): 181 mg
Cottage cheese, 1% milk fat (1 cup): 138 mg
Tofu, soft with calcium sulfate* (1/2 cup): 138 mg
Instant breakfast drink mix (8 ounces): 105–250 mg
Frozen yogurt, vanilla, soft serve (1/2 cup): 103 mg
Cold cereal, calcium-fortified (1/2 cup): 100–1,000 mg
Turnip greens, fresh, boiled (1/2 cup): 99 mg
Kale, fresh, cooked (1/2 cup): 94 mg
Kale, raw, chopped (1 cup): 90 mg
Ice cream, vanilla (1 cup): 84 mg
Soy drink, calcium-fortified (1/2 cup): 80–500 mg
Chinese cabbage, raw, shredded (1 cup): 74 mg
Bread, white (1 slice): 73 mg

Pudding, chocolate (4 ounces): 55 mg
Tortilla, corn (1 - 6″ diameter) : 46 mg
Tortilla, flour (1 - 6″ diameter): 32 mg
Sour cream, reduced fat (2 tablespoons): 31 mg
Bread, whole-wheat (1 slice): 30 mg
Broccoli, raw (1/2 cup): 21 mg
Cheese, cream, regular (1 tablespoon): 14 mg

Appendix A.5: Vitamin D Rich Foods

Food (Portion Size): Vitamin D

Salmon, sockeye (3 ounces): 19.8 mcg

Salmon, smoked (3 ounces): 14.5 mcg

Salmon, canned (3 ounces): 11.6 mcg

Rockfish, cooked (3 ounces): 6.5 mcg

Tuna, light, canned in oil (3 ounces): 5.7 mcg

Sardine, canned in oil (3 ounces): 4.1 mcg

Tuna, canned in water (3 ounces): 3.8 mcg

Orange juice (1 cup) 3.4 mcg

Whole milk (1 cup) 3.2 mcg

Whole chocolate milk (1 cup) 3.2 mcg

2% chocolate milk (1 cup) 3 mcg

Milk (nonfat, 1% and 2%) (1 cup) 2.9 mcg

Low-fat chocolate milk (1%) (1 cup) 2.8 mcg

Soymilk (1 cup) 2.7 mcg

Evaporated milk, nonfat (1/2 cup) 2.6 mcg

Flatfish (flounder & sole) (3 ounces) 2.5 mcg

Fortified cereals (3/4–1 1/4 cup): 0.9–2.5 mcg

Rice drink (1 cup): 2.4 mcg

Herring, pickled (3 ounces): 2.4 mcg

Pork, cooked (3 ounces): 0.6–2.2 mcg

Cod, cooked (3 ounces): 1 mcg

Beef liver, cooked (3 ounces): 1 mcg

Cured ham (3 ounces): 0.6–0.8 mcg

Egg, hard-boiled (1 large) 0.7 mcg

Shiitake mushrooms (1/2 cup) 0.6 mcg

Canadian bacon (2 slices): 0.5 mcg

1 mcg of vitamin D is equivalent to 40 IU

Appendix A.6: DHA and EPA Food Sources

FOOD

Salmon, Atlantic, farmed and wild
Canned salmon
Herring
Sardines
Mackerel
Trout
Oysters
Sea bass
Shrimp
Lobster
Tuna, light, canned in water
Scallops
Cod, Pacific
Tuna, yellowfin
*Fortified eggs
Chicken breast
*Fortified milk

(*DHA only)

Appendix A.7: Fiber-Rich Foods

Food (Portion Size): Fiber content

Beans, cooked (1/2 cup): 6–10 g
Bran ready-to-eat cereal (100%) (1/3 cup): 9.1 g
Split peas, lentils, chickpeas (1/2 cup): 5–8 g
Artichoke, cooked (1/2 cup hearts): 7.2 g
Pear (1 medium): 5.5 g
Soybeans, mature, cooked (1/2 cup): 5.2 g
Plain rye wafer crackers (2 wafers): 5 g
Bran ready-to-eat cereals (1/3–3/4 cup): 2–5 g
Asian pear (1 small): 4.4 g
Whole-wheat English muffin (1 muffin): 4.4 g
Bulgur, cooked (1/2 cup): 4.1 g
Mixed vegetables, cooked (1/2 cup): 4 g
Raspberries (1/2 cup): 4 g
Green peas, cooked (1/2 cup): 3–4 g
Sweet potato, baked in skin (1 medium): 3.8 g
Blackberries (1/2 cup): 3.8 g
Soybeans, green, cooked (1/2 cup): 3.8 g
Prunes, stewed (1/2 cup): 3.8 g
Shredded wheat cereal (1/2 cup): 2–4 g
Figs, dried (1/4 cup): 3.7 g
Apple, with skin (1 small): 3.6 g
Pumpkin, canned (1/2 cup): 3.6 g
Greens (spinach, collards) (1/2 cup): 2–3 g
Almonds (1 ounce): 3.5 g
Sauerkraut, canned (1/2 cup): 3.4 g
Whole wheat spaghetti, cooked (1/2 cup): 3.1 g
Banana (1 medium): 3.1 g
Orange (1 medium): 3.1 g
Guava (1 fruit): 3 g

Potato, baked, with skin (1 small): 3 g
Oat bran muffin (1 small): 3 g
Pearled barley, cooked (1/2 cup): 3 g
Dates (1/4 cup): 2.9 g
Winter squash, cooked (1/2 cup): 2.9 g
Parsnips, cooked (1/2 cup): 2.8 g

Appendix B: Recipes

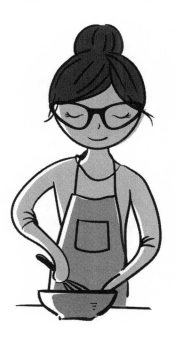

Appendix B.1: Straightforward, You Do It Recipes

Basic Fruit Smoothie

I've used smoothies as an after-school snack for years. This is my basic recipe; however, I mix and match ingredients (especially fruit) more than not.

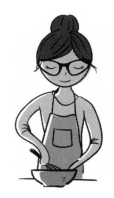

Ingredients:

1 cup milk
½ cup plain or flavored yogurt
½ cup 100% juice
1 cup frozen fruit
1 to 2 tablespoons honey, maple syrup, or agave

Directions:

In a blender, add milk, juice, yogurt and frozen fruit. Blend on high until completely mixed and smooth. Add honey or other sweetener to taste and blend for 5 seconds. Makes 2 servings.

Smoothie Bowls

I like the Minimalist Baker's version of a smoothie bowl, and it's all about the blending. Remember nice cream? Well, it's the backbone of this smoothie bowl. You can find her original recipe here: https://minimalistbaker.com/favorite-smoothie-bowl-5-minutes/

Ingredients:

1 small frozen banana, sliced
   1 cup frozen mixed berries
   2 to 3 tablespoons milk (or non-dairy substitute)

Toppings (optional combinations):

1 tablespoon seeds (pumpkin, hemp, chia, or other)
   2 tablespoons granola
   1 tablespoon unsweetened coconut
   1 tablespoon nut butter
   Sliced fresh fruit

Directions:

Add the frozen banana and berries to the blender and process on low until pulverized. Scrape down the sides. Add the milk and blend on low until it looks creamy and mimics soft-serve ice cream. Transfer to two bowls and decorate with desired toppings.

English Muffin Pizza

A super simple, easy snack that will excite
and satisfy many kids.

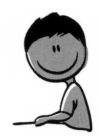

Ingredients:

½ English muffin
    1 to 2 tablespoons spaghetti sauce
    1 to 2 tablespoons low-fat mozzarella cheese
    Turkey pepperoni slices (optional)

Directions:

If using an oven or toaster oven, pre-heat to 400 F. Spoon tomato
sauce onto the inside of an English muffin and spread evenly
with the back of a spoon. Sprinkle cheese on top and add
pepperoni slices if desired. Toast in the toaster oven, or bake in
the oven, at 400 F until cheese is bubbly.

Walk with Me Taco Packets

My old pool association used to serve these, and my kids loved them. They are a 'build-your-own' concept with a smorgasbord presentation. The best part? You can make these heartier with ground chicken or beans and serve them as a main meal.

Ingredients:

6 individual bags Sun Chips (original or garden salsa flavor)
    Shredded lettuce
    Diced tomato
    Corn
    Salsa
    Reduced fat (2%) shredded Mexican cheese
    Diced avocado
    Reduced-fat sour cream (optional)

Directions:

Gently crush each bag of chips. Cut the bags lengthwise with scissors. Prepare bowls of lettuce, chopped tomatoes, corn, shredded cheese, diced avocado, salsa, and any other desired toppings. Let your child top his chips with his preference of toppings.

Baked Tater Skins

On a chilly day, these can be a welcoming twist from the usual packaged snack. The microwave helps speed up the process, but you can use the oven instead if you prefer.

Ingredients:

2 medium potatoes
 4 tablespoons shredded cheddar cheese
 Bacon bits
 Low-fat sour cream (optional)

Directions:

Pre-heat oven or toaster oven to 350 F. Pierce the skin of the potatoes with a fork and microwave them on the "potato" setting, or for 4 to 5 minutes. Test with a fork to make sure they're done. Let cool. Cut in half length-wise and spoon out the flesh. (You can save this for a quick mashed potato side dish later, or serve it alongside the tater skins.) Place the hollowed-out skins on a cookie sheet that's been prepped with non-stick cooking spray. Fill the interior of the skins with 1 tablespoon of cheese. Bake for 7 to 8 minutes or until cheese is melted. Remove from the oven and sprinkle with bacon bits. Top with sour cream if desired. Makes 4 skins.

Quick Quesadillas

Ingredients:

1 flour tortilla, burrito-size
3 tablespoons Mexican-style shredded cheese

Directions:

Place the flour tortilla on a microwave-safe plate. Spread shredded cheese evenly over the entire tortilla. Microwave for 1 minute. Remove and fold the tortilla in half; cut into 4 to 6 wedges.

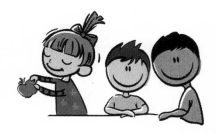

Appendix B.2: Healthier Homemade Snacks

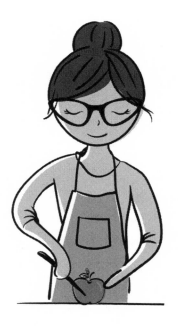

Easy Stove-Top Granola

You don't have to turn the oven on with this recipe!

Ingredients:

¼ cup canola oil
    3 cups oatmeal
    1/3 cup brown sugar
    ¼ cup honey
    ½ teaspoon cinnamon
    1 teaspoon imitation butter flavoring
    a pinch of Kosher salt
    ¼ cup peanuts
    ¼ cup flaked coconut
    ¼ cup mini chocolate chips

Directions:

In a large non-stick skillet over medium heat, toast oats for 10-15 minutes, or until light brown and crispy.

Add sugar, honey, cinnamon, butter flavoring, and salt, stirring to coat the oats. (Note: If you have a gas stove, lower the heat. If you have an electric stove, remove the skillet from the burner while adding these ingredients.)

Place the skillet back on low heat to ensure oats are coated and sugar is melted, stirring constantly for about 2-3 minutes; granola will brown and bubble up.

Remove from the heat and place granola on a cookie sheet to cool.

Once cool, add peanuts, coconut and chocolate chips.

Store in an airtight container or Ziploc bag for up to a week. (It won't last that long, guaranteed!)

GORP (Trail Mix)

Heading to a day at the beach or pool? Off to a sporting event? Or just need a grab-and-go snack that hits all the nutrition highlights? GORP is your friend and answer.

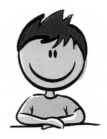

Ingredients:

1 box oatmeal squares cereal (or other squarish cereal)
    2 cups lightly salted peanuts (1 container)
    2 cups raisins (or other dried fruit)
    1, 16-ounce bag waffle pretzels
    2 cups (or more or less) plain chocolate M & M's

Directions:

Mix all ingredients in a large bowl. Store in a large Ziploc bag or airtight plastic container or package into individual baggies.

Almond Granola Bars by Rebecca Bitzer & Associates (@marylanddietitians)

Almond Granola Bars Recipe is a dietitian-approved quick snack loaded with fiber and healthy unsaturated fats and so easy to prepare. Also gluten-free, vegetarian, budget friendly, and kid friendly.

Ingredients:

1 cup pitted dates
   1 cup almonds chopped
   1 1/2 cup oats
   1/4 cup honey
   1/4 cup Justin's Honey Almond Butter

Instructions:

1. Place dates in a food processor. Blend well (mixture may form a ball, or several balls).

2. Combine dates, almonds, and oats in a bowl. Set aside.

3. Heat honey and almond butter on low until melted. Pour into dates, almonds, and oats bowl. Mix well, breaking up the dates. Spray your hands with some cooking spray and use your hands to mix once the mixture has cooled.

4. Spray an 8x8 pan with cooking spray. Spray the bottom of a flat, sturdy drinking class with cooking spray. Pour the mixture into the pan and then press down with the bottom of the glass until everything is compact.

5. Chill in the fridge for 30 minutes.

6. Cut the bars into 10 pieces.

Visit www.rbitzer.com

Strawberry Kiwi Fruit Leather by Dana Angelo White (@dana_angelo_white)

Commercially prepared fruit leathers are filled with highly processed sweeteners and even trans fats! This recipe keeps the sugar content in check.

Ingredients:

1 ½ cups chopped fresh strawberries
½ cup chopped fresh kiwi
2 tablespoons sugar
2 tablespoons honey

Instructions:

1. Preheat oven to 170°F.
2. Line a baking sheet with parchment paper or a Silpat mat and set aside.
3. Place fruit, honey, and sugar in a medium saucepan. Bring to a boil and cook for about 5 minutes, then puree using an immersion blender.* Continue to cook over medium-high heat for an additional 10 to 15 minutes or until syrupy; the mixture should be thick enough to coat the back of a spoon.
4. Pour the hot fruit mixture onto prepared baking sheet and spread evenly into approximately an 8 × 12-inch rectangle.
5. Place in the oven and bake for 3 hours. After 3 hours, turn off the oven and allow to sit overnight.
6. Cut into strips with a pizza cutter; roll up in a clean piece of parchment paper.
7. Store in an airtight container for up to 3 weeks.

*If you do not have an immersion blender, puree in a food processor and then return mixture to saucepan.

Yield: 12 strips

Visit www.danawhitenutrition.com

Double Chocolate Brownies by Jodi Danen, RD (@CreateKidsClub)

These Double Chocolate Brownies are so good it's hard to just have one. They are oil free and contain no flour. Make them once and you'll see how many rave reviews they receive!

Ingredients:

15 oz. can black beans drained and rinsed

2-3 tbsp. water

3 large eggs

3 tbsps. unsweetened applesauce

3/4 cup granulated sugar

1/2 cup cocoa powder

1/2 cup mini semi-sweet chocolate chips + extra for sprinkling on top

1 tsp. vanilla extract

1/2 tsp. baking soda

1/2 tsp. salt

Instructions:

1. Preheat oven to 350 degrees.

2. Prepare 8 x 8-inch baking dish with non-stick cooking spray.

3. Add drained black beans plus 2 tbsp. water to blender. Puree until smooth. Add additional tbsp. of water if the beans are still too thick to puree. Scrape sides to ensure it purees all beans.

4. Add the rest of the ingredients to blender, blending until well mixed.

5. Pour mixture into prepared baking dish.

6. Bake 30 minutes or until knife inserted into center of pan comes out clean.

Visit www.createkidsclub.com

Easy, Healthy Avocado Brownies by Megan Byrd, RD (@theoregondietitian)

These healthy avocado brownies are so easy to make! With heart-healthy ingredients, this simple vegan brownie recipe turns out fudgy and delicious!

Ingredients:

¼ cup avocado, mashed
   ¼ cup avocado oil
   ¼ cup cold brew coffee
   ¼ cup water
   ½ cup maple syrup
   1 cup whole wheat pastry flour
   ½ cup cocoa powder
   1 tsp baking soda
   2 tbsp ground flax
   ½ tsp salt
   1 cup vegan chocolate chips (divided)

Instructions:

1. Preheat oven to 350°.

2. Mix the first 5 ingredients in a medium bowl. Set aside.

3. In another medium bowl, mix the dry ingredients and ½ cup of the chocolate chips.

4. Add the wet ingredients into the dry ingredients and stir until well combined.

5. Grease a 9×9 baking pan, and pour the batter into the pan, smoothing evenly. Sprinkle the remaining ½ cup of chocolate chips on top of the batter.

6. Bake at 350° for 14-15 minutes for a fudgy texture, or 16-17 minutes for a cake-like texture.

Visit www.theoregondietitian.com

No Added Sugar Chocolate Oatmeal Cookies by Shahzadi Devje, RD (@desiliciousrd)

Probably one of the easiest, healthiest, and most delicious Chocolate Oatmeal Cookies you'll ever make. Rolled oats, ripe bananas, dates, cacao, and cinnamon come together to create an incredibly soft, unbelievably chewy, and absolutely wholesome cookie recipe.

Ingredients:

3 bananas (large, ripe)
    1 cup dates (pitted, soft)
    1/4 cup coconut oil (organic, cold-pressed)
    1/2 tsp cinnamon powder
    1/4 tsp baking powder
    salt (pinch)
    1 tbsp cocoa powder, unsweetened
    2 cups rolled oats
    1 tbsp cacao nibs, unsweetened

Instructions:

1. Preheat oven to 350 degrees F (175 degrees C).
2. Line the baking tray with parchment paper.
3. Blend all the ingredients (save half the oats and stir into the blended mixture).
4. Spoon out on the parchment-lined baking tray. The cookies should be about two inches apart.
5. Sprinkle with cacao nibs.
6. Bake in the oven on the middle/high shelf for 10 mins. Rotate the tray and bake for an additional 5 mins.

7. Let them sit on the hot baking sheet for five minutes before serving.

Visit www.shahzadidevje.com

No-Bake Peanut Butter Oatmeal Protein Balls by Lauren Sharifi, MPH, RD (@laurensharifird)

These No-Bake Peanut Butter Oatmeal Protein Balls are a nutrient-packed snack that will help keep your and your kids' taste buds and stomachs satisfied!

Ingredients:

1 cup old-fashioned oats
    1 cup cereal (e.g., Cheerios or Corn Flakes)
    1/3 cup nuts
    1/3 cup dried fruit
    1/4 cup semi-sweet chocolate chips
    2 tablespoons chia and/or hemp seeds
    1 teaspoon cinnamon
    1/2 cup natural nut or seed butter
    1/4 cup honey

Instructions:

1. In a large bowl add oats, cereal, nuts, seeds, dried fruit, chocolate chips, and cinnamon. Mix.

2. In a small bowl, add peanut butter and honey. If needed, heat for 30 seconds to make it easier to mix.

3. Add peanut butter and honey mixture to dry mixture and mix to combine.

4. Using a small cookie scoop or spoon, mash mixture together to break cereal and nuts into smaller pieces. (This makes it easier to form mixture into balls.) Then using the scoop or spoon portion out ~ 1/8 cup of granola mixture and form into a ball. To prevent the mixture from sticking to your hands, try

spraying a small amount of cooking spray and rubbing over your hands (you may need to repeat every few balls).

5. Place formed balls on a cookie sheet or plate and place cookie sheet in freezer for 10 minutes to allow granola balls to harden.

6. Store granola balls in an airtight container or plastic bag in the refrigerator.

Visit www.laurensharifi.com

Giant Oatmeal, Banana, Peanut Butter Breakfast Cookies by Sarah Gold, RD (@busy.mom.nutrition)

Filled with wholesome ingredients like oats, nut butter, bananas, and flaxseeds, with very little added sugar, these hearty cookies are healthy enough to enjoy for breakfast or as an afternoon pick-me-up, yet so delicious you'll also want to eat them as an after-dinner treat.

Ingredients:

1 large overripe banana, mashed
    2 eggs
    2 Tbsp ground flax
    1/4 cup maple syrup
    1 tsp vanilla extract
    3 1/2 cups rolled oats
    1 cup peanut butter
    1 tsp baking soda
    2/3 cup chocolate chips

Instructions:

1. Preheat oven to 350F.

2. Beat banana, eggs, flax, maple syrup, and vanilla until well blended.

3. Stir in oats, peanut butter, and baking soda until mixed. Stir in chocolate chips until evenly distributed through batter. Do not over mix.

4. Using a 1/4 cup measuring cup, scoop a heaping scoop of the batter onto a parchment-lined (or use a baking mat) baking sheet. Flatten the cookies down a bit with the back of the

measuring cup. For smaller cookies, fill only half the measuring cup or use a heaping tablespoon.

5. Bake for 12-14 minutes, until cookies get a golden-brown edge. Smaller cookies will need less baking time, so check after about 9-10 minutes.

6. Remove from baking sheet and let cool on wire cooling rack.

7. Store in an airtight container on the counter for up to 3 days or in freezer for up to 2 months.

Visit www.sarahgoldrd.com

Peace Popcorn by **Laura McCann, RD** (**@myfamilyfork**)

This healthy, fiber-rich snack can be addictive! It's packed with B-vitamins, including B12, from the nutritional yeast, and naturally occurring iodine in the sea vegetables (kelp or dulse). Popcorn is a great snack to go for when you're feeling the munchies and want to indulge in a larger portion.

Ingredients:

    1/4 cup popcorn kernels

    1/4 teaspoons Bragg's Liquid Aminos spray

    4 Tablespoons Nutritional/Brewer's Yeast

    1 teaspoon Dulse or Kelp flakes

    1/2 teaspoon black pepper freshly ground

Instructions:

1. Pop popcorn in an air popper.*

2. Spray with Bragg's Liquid Aminos.

3. Sprinkle generously with nutritional yeast.

4. Shake dulse flakes over popcorn, followed by a few cranks of freshly ground black pepper.

*Don't have an air popper? You can also pop your popcorn in a pot on the stove, then add toppings.

Visit www.myfamilyfork.com

Strawberry-Banana Chickpea Flour Muffins by Sarah Schlicter, RD (@bucketlisttummy)

Strawberry-Banana Chickpea Flour Muffins are fluffy, yet high in protein. These easy, gluten-free muffins are ready in 30 minutes and are perfect for on-the-go snacks for kids.

Ingredients:

1 cup chickpea flour
1/2 cup oat flour
1 tsp baking soda
¼ tsp salt
½ tsp cinnamon
¼ cup brown sugar or coconut sugar
3 medium, ripe bananas, mashed (Do you mean medium-ripe bananas, OR medium (size), ripe bananas?)
2 large eggs
1 tsp apple cider vinegar
2 tsp vanilla extract
2 tbsp coconut oil, melted and cooled (or butter)
1 cup strawberries, diced (about 6-7 large strawberries)

Instructions:

1. Preheat oven to 375.
2. In a medium bowl, combine all dry ingredients (chickpea flour through brown sugar).
3. In a large bowl, combine mashed bananas, eggs, vinegar, vanilla, and butter.
4. Pour dry ingredients into wet ingredients and stir until combined and moistened.
5. Last, fold in the strawberries (or any berries of choice)

6. Pour batter into a greased muffin tin.

7. Bake for 16-20 minutes, or until tops are set, browned, and a toothpick comes out clean.

Let cool on a wire rack before enjoying!

Visit www.bucketlisttummy.com

Edible Chocolate Chip Cookie Dough by Holley Grainger, RD (@holleygrainger)

Our healthy, edible cookie dough featuring chickpeas and graham cracker crumbs won with taste testers hands down.

Ingredients:

1 cup graham cracker crumbs (about 7 graham cracker sheets) *see note below
    1 can chickpeas, drained, rinsed, and patted dry
    1/4 cup nut butter (preferably unsweetened)
    1/4 cup brown sugar
    1 Tbsp vanilla extract
    1/4 tsp salt
    2 Tbsp milk (if needed)
    1/3 cup mini chocolate chips

Instructions:

1. Add graham cracker crumbs (pulse graham crackers in a food processor to make a fine crumb), chickpeas, nut butter, brown sugar, vanilla, and salt in a food processor.

2. Blend until smooth. If needed, add milk until it reaches desired consistency.

3. Remove blade from food processor and transfer cookie dough mixture into a medium bowl.

4. Gently stir in chocolate chips.

5. Press plastic wrap firmly on top of cookie dough and refrigerate at least 1 hour.

6. To serve, remove plastic wrap and serve cookie dough as a dip, roll into balls, or eat with a spoon!

Visit www.holleygrainger.com

Creamy Chocolate Peanut Butter "Ice Cream" by Liz Ward (@betteristhenewperfect)

This dairy-free vegan "ice cream" is delicious and offers a serving of fruit, too!

Ingredients:
_____

2 medium ripe bananas, cut into chunks and frozen (Freeze for at least 2 hours.)

   2 Tbsp. peanut butter (with no added sugar, if desired)

   2 Tbsp. unsweetened cocoa powder

   1/2 tsp. pure vanilla extract

   2 Tbsp. chopped peanuts

Instructions:
_____

1. Place bananas in a large food processor.

   2. Add the peanut butter, cocoa powder, and vanilla.

   3. Blend until smooth, about 2 to 3 minutes.

   4. Transfer to serving bowls and garnish with peanuts. Serve immediately.

Visit www.betteristhenewperfect.com

Appendix C: Packaged To-Go Snack Ideas

Planters NUT-rition Heart Healthy Mix
Biena Chickpea Snacks
Hippeas Organic Chickpea Snacks
Puffins Cereal
Annie's Whole Wheat Bunnies
Wholly Guacamole
Kind Healthy Grains Bar
Boom Chicka Pop
Stoneyfield Whole Milk Yogurt Squeezie
Sabra Hummus Cups
Skinny Pop Popcorn Cakes
Blue Diamond Almonds 100-Calorie Pack
365 Reduced Fat Popcorn
Simple Mills Almond Flour Crackers
Sellon Farms Pistachio Chewy Bites
Kind Nut Butter Bars
Rhythm Superfoods Beet Chips
Horizon Organic Good & Go!
Yumbutter
Mini Kefir by Lifeway
Quaker Breakfast Flats
Triscuit Reduced Fat Crackers
Kind Pressed Fruit and Chia Bars
Bare Apple Chips
Rx Bars (any flavor)
Turkey Jerky
Frigo String Cheese
Beanitos Bean Chips
Justin's Peanut Butter Single Packs
Raisins
Yogurt-covered Raisins

Made Good Bars
Brainiac Yogurt Sticks
Brainiac Applesauce Pouch
Funny Face Dried Cranberries
PopCorners Sea Salt Chips
Babybel Mini Cheese Wheels
Saffron Road Roasted Chickpeas
Seapoint Farms Dry Roasted Edamame
Ritz Bits

Appendix D: Easy Nutritious Snack Combos

Shredded wheat, low fat milk, and blueberries
Layered yogurt, granola, and strawberries
Skewered cantaloupe and cheddar cheese cubes
Apple and cheese slices
Banana dipped in peanut butter
Strawberries dipped in low fat strawberry cream cheese and then in granola
Clementine and a cheese stick
Applesauce cup and graham crackers
Hummus and flat pretzels
Hummus and baby carrots
Tortilla with melted cheese (quesadilla)
Baked potato with shredded Monterey Jack cheese and salsa
Air popped popcorn and hot chocolate (made with low fat milk)
Whole wheat toast with butter and jam
Toasted oat bread with nut butter and banana slices
English muffin with butter and honey
Banana or other fruited muffin and 6 oz. milk
Deli meat wrapped around a cheese stick
Sugar snap peas and red peppers with Laughing Cow cheese
Coconut yogurt and mini chocolate chips
Nuts and dried fruit
Diced tomato and cottage cheese
Oatmeal cookies and milk
100% Orange Juice + Yogurt blended and frozen into a popsicle
Half of a sandwich and ½ cup of 100% fruit juice
Cheese and crackers
Peanut butter and pretzels
Mini bagel and cream cheese
Homemade trail mix (cereal, nuts, and dried fruit)
Red grapes and cheese kabobs

Pepperoni mini pizza (pita bread, tomato sauce, cheese and turkey pepperoni slices)

Black olives, feta cheese and pita bread

Frozen yogurt with fresh berries

All fruit popsicle and roasted almonds

Instant oatmeal, slivered almonds and berries

Low fat chocolate milk and whole grain crackers

Mozzarella and tomato skewers

Tuna fish salad and whole grain crackers

Chicken salad and green grapes

Tossed salad with cheese cubes and dressing

Low fat Ranch dressing and veggies

Smoothie made with frozen berries, yogurt and 100% juice

Celery sticks with cream cheese or nut butter

Chocolate hazelnut butter and graham crackers

Melon balls with a dollop of Greek Yogurt (cantaloupe, honeydew)

Mashed avocado spread on whole grain crackers

Whole grain waffle swiped with peanut butter

1/2 grilled cheese sandwich and 100% vegetable juice (i.e., V-8)

Baked potato and cottage cheese

Toast with peanut butter

Pita bread and hummus

Nut-based or protein-rich granola bar

Pretzels and dried cherries mix

Raisins and peanuts

Mini bagel with jam

Beef jerky and a mozzarella cheese stick

Hard-boiled egg and half an English muffin

String cheese and snow peas

Whole grain blueberry muffin (regular size) and ½ cup of milk or soy milk